Arrived Too Soon

The Essential Guide For
Parents With Premmies

Dr. R. Kishore Kumar

STARDOM BOOKS

WORLDWIDE

www.StardomBooks.com

STARDOM BOOKS

A Division of Stardom Publishing

and infoYOGIS Technologies.

105-501 Silverside Road

Wilmington, DE 19809

SECOND EDITION NOVEMBER 2020

Stardom Books

ARRIVED TOO SOON /
The Essential Guide for Parents with Premmies.

Dr. R. KISHORE KUMAR

p. 104
cm. 13.5 X 21.5

Category: Parenting

ISBN-13: 978-1-7332116-4-2

FOREWORD

You have just experienced a wonderful miracle - the birth of your baby. Your miracle, however, arrived earlier than you expected - maybe weeks or even months earlier. Your baby is now being cared for in a Neonatal Intensive Care Unit (NICU). You probably are overwhelmed right now and have a lot of questions regarding your baby's health. For instance, when he/she will get to go home, and how you are going to cope with this unexpected situation.

This book has been prepared to answer some of the common concerns which most parents have. Although it is not easy, but try your best not to worry; we know you may feel completely helpless. But you can rest assured knowing that while your baby is in Cloudnine, he/she will get the best medical care available. Cloudnine has one of the highest survival rates of preterm babies in the world so far, due to its international standard of care. Do not hesitate to discuss any question you may have with the NICU staff. Let them know if you are scared or confused. Helping parents like you deal with their fears, feelings, and frustrations is an important part of their job.

This book has been planned for quite some time, the global action report on preterm birth 'Born Too Soon' provided us the first global estimate of preterm birth. The report shows the extent to which preterm birth is on the rise, and that it is now the second leading cause of death globally for children under five, after pneumonia. This hastened our efforts and resulted in the first edition, but now we are preparing this second edition after 7 years of various feedbacks from parents like you. Simultaneously, taking a cue from 'Born Too Soon', the Indian Foundation for Premature

Babies (IFPB) have prepared a sequel on Preterm Birth in India. Neonatologists from across the country, including experts from Cloudnine, have contributed data and content on various issues related to India's preterm births in the report 'Delivered Too Soon - India Story' which was released recently.

I heartily thank Shri. U. T. Khader, Honourable Minister for Health and Family Welfare, Government of Karnataka, under whose august aegis the first edition of "Arrived Too Soon" was launched. I also thank Dr. Arvind Shenoi, my colleague, for giving constructive suggestions and writing the preface for this first edition; Dr. Chitra Shankar for writing the section on follow up of preterm babies and all my other neonatal colleagues Dr. Nandini Nagar & Dr. S. V. Girish- for providing valuable insights.

We will constantly strive to improve our book, as with our services, so if you feel there is something we could have written better or could have added, or even deleted, please let us know. We will include your suggestions and comments in the next edition to make things better!

Wishing you a stress free and successful experience

Regards
Kishore

Prof. Dr. R. Kishore Kumar
MMBS, DCH, (Mys), MD (Paed Gold Medalist), DCH (Lond), MRCP (Paed), FRCPCH (UK), FRCPI, FRACP (Australia), FNNF, FIAP, MHCD (Harvard)
Senior Consultant Neonatologist &Paediatrician, Cloudnine Hospital, Chairman & Managing Director Cloudnine Hospitals India Adjunct Professor of Neonatology, Notre Dame University, Perth, Australia
1533, 9th Main, 3rd Block, Jayanagar, Bangalore 560 011, India
Tel: +91 80 4020 2222 Fax: +91 80 4020 2233
Email: drkishore@cloudninecare.com

CONTENTS

PREFACE

It gives me great pleasure to write this preface to the first edition of the premmie baby book. This book is the result of the seminal work put in by Dr. R. Kishore Kumar in compiling various important bits of information sought by parents of premature babies.

The story of Gautam Buddha reminds us of the importance of working towards saving small and fragile premature newborns. Legend has it that when Princess Mahamaya was traveling to her father's residence she delivered a small baby in the gardens of Lumbini. The infant was so frail that it took a renowned seer to convince the father and the king that this frail infant would one day be a leader of men. History stands witness to the world-shaking contributions made by this premature neonate. We as neonatologists dedicate our lives to saving these small infants who have the potential of contributing greatly to the development of the human race. The initial steps in the journey of a premature baby can have many potential problems. This book will hopefully act as a guidepost to parents traversing this journey.

This book runs in two parts. The first part talks about some of the various illnesses that afflict premature babies and the second is like a manual for follow up. The second part will be useful once the baby is discharged from NICU. It needs to be brought in for each neuro-developmental visit, which are planned at discharge, as well as eye exam, etc.

The highlight of this book is that it talks about the equipment, people and also about the aspects of NICU that worry parents who visit and find their fragile newborn there. However, no manual or book can be all-encompassing. Hence, feel free to interact with the staff and ask them questions about anything you want to know. The best option is to discuss all this with the neonatologist who counsels you every morning.

The book underlines the Cloudnine philosophy of partnering with parents and making even a premature delivery an enjoyable experience, and as stress-free as possible. We hope the parents find this book a useful companion to their journey through our NICU and beyond.

Dr. Arvind Shenoi

MBBS, MD, DM (Neonatology PGI), Fellowship in NICU (Australia) Senior Consultant Neonatologist & Medical Director Cloudnine Hospital, Old Airport Road, Bangalore

INTRODUCTION

Every year some babies are born prematurely (preterm birth) i.e. born at 37/40 weeks or even earlier. Even though you try not to, you may end up asking yourself, Why me? Is this my fault? If you are feeling this way, you are not alone because not all pregnancies go smoothly. We have developed this book to address some common questions parents have regarding preterm delivery.

Remember that each woman, each baby, each pregnancy and each delivery is completely unique. Your paediatrician is always the best source for answering questions about your own unique experience.

Some commonly asked questions

Q: What causes preterm delivery? Can this happen to me again?

A: Approximately half of all women who give birth prematurely go into preterm labour for unknown reasons. The remainder have medical conditions such as toxemia,

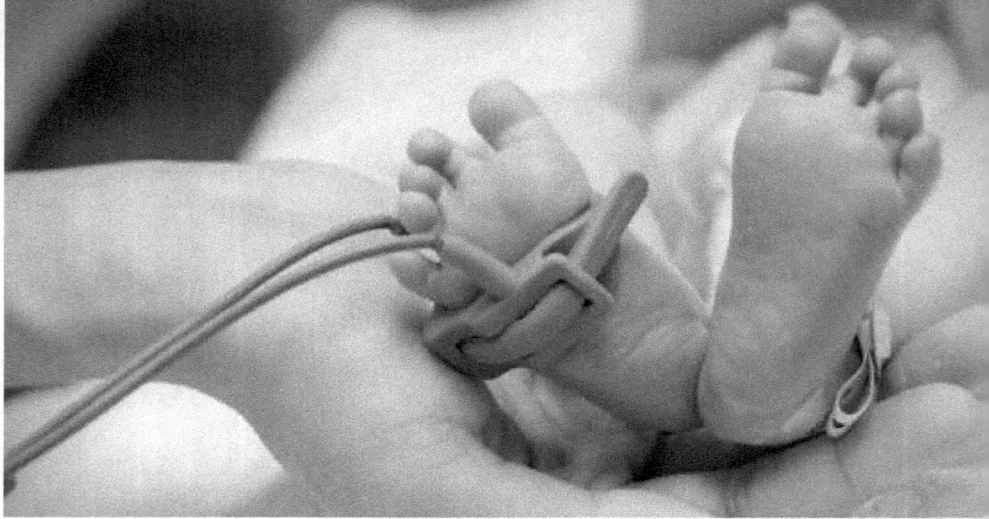

incompetent cervix, placenta praevia, etc., which can often result in preterm delivery. Statistically, a woman who has had a preterm baby runs a 25% to 50% chance of having another one. Although for many women, preterm delivery is a one-time event in their childbearing history.

Q: Is it my fault that my baby was born prematurely?

A: It is neither yours nor anyone else's fault that your baby was born early. So don't blame yourself. Some conditions like maternal high blood pressure can cause premature delivery. But some other factors involve the baby. Twins and other multiple births are often born too early. Babies with congenital defects, or abnormally positioned placenta are also often born prematurely. Remember, your pediatrician is your best source for information about your individual delivery.

Q: I went into labor prematurely. No one can explain why it happened. Does anyone know what causes preterm labor?

A: Preterm labor can begin painlessly and may be mistaken for the Braxton-Hicks contractions (false labour pains), which most women experience during pregnancy. Unlike Braxton-Hicks contractions, real labor contractions occur at fairly regular intervals and cause the cervix to shorten (efface) and open (dilate). No one knows what causes full-term labor till now, so it's impossible to say for sure why it begins prematurely. However, researchers are investigating the hormones during pregnancy to see whether abnormal levels of these substances (hormones) may be involved.

Q: I was told I had an incompetent cervix. What does this mean? Is there a way to correct this problem?

A: Incompetent cervix is the term used for a cervix that opens, often painlessly, in mid- pregnancy leading to a miscarriage or preterm birth. This condition usually results from damages to the connective tissue of the cervix during previous births, or surgery involving the cervix. It can also be caused by diethylstilbestrol (DES) exposure. Many DES daughters (daughters of women given the drug diethylstilbestrol during their pregnancies in the 1940s and 1950s) have had abnormalities of the cervix and uterus, which made it difficult for them to carry a baby to full term. An incompetent cervix can sometimes be reinforced by a procedure called en-circlage. During this procedure the cervix is stitched shut early in pregnancy. The stitches are removed before the baby is born. Since cervical en-circlage does carry risks (the possibility of infection and even the stimulation of preterm labor) some doctors may be hesitant to perform this procedure, unless they feel absolutely sure that the problem is actually an incompetent cervix. A reliable diagnosis may be difficult to make, since a normal cervix can also open early as the result of undetected preterm labor.

Q: I felt fine until my sixth month of pregnancy. Then I developed toxemia. What causes it?

A: Toxemia is a condition affecting 5% to 7% of all pregnant women. The first stage of toxemia is called pre-eclampsia. It is characterized by high blood pressure, protein in the urine and rapid weight gain due to fluid retention. If left untreated, it can develop into eclampsia - a severe form of toxemia. Its symptoms sometimes can include convulsions, brain hemorrhage and coma. Because toxemia often involves reduction in blood flow to the fetus, the baby may be smaller than normal for the baby's gestational age. Bed rest, nutritious, diet, and blood pressure medication can sometimes manage toxemia. When these measures fail, preterm delivery is necessary to save the mother and baby. Toxemia usually occurs in first-time pregnancies.

Q: Can illness during pregnancy cause preterm delivery?

A: A mother's general health before and during pregnancy can affect the outcome. Pre-existing illnesses such as diabetes, kidney disease, high blood pressure and sickle cell anemia do increase the chance of preterm delivery.

Preterm birth can also be the result of an illness in the unborn baby. Although the membranes and placenta provide a barrier against many infections, certain organisms are still able to cross the placenta or enter the womb, possibly through weak spots in the membranes. An infected baby may be born to a mother who has had only mild symptoms of illness or no symptoms at all. Why some babies become infected while others do not is not well understood.

Q: Can sex during pregnancy cause prematurity?

A: A study of close to 11,000 pregnancies revealed no difference in the incidence of preterm rupture of the membranes, intrauterine infection or prematurity among women who engaged in intercourse throughout their pregnancy from those who did not. However, sexual activity may release oxytocin, a hormone that stimulates uterine contractions. For a woman already beginning labor, sexual activity might speed things along. This is why doctors recommend that women abstain from these activities if they show actual signs or symptoms of preterm labor.

Q: I did everything right during my pregnancy. A friend was pregnant at the same time.

She lived on diet soda, smoked cigarettes, and drank alcohol. She had a healthy nine-pound baby. I had a two-pound premature baby. Why me?

A: Statistically, women who eat well avoid harmful substances and get good prenatal care, do have better pregnancy outcomes than those who do not. However, there are always exceptions. Women who do all the wrong things can still have healthy full-term babies, and women who do everything right can still have preterm babies.

YOUR PRETERM BABY

If your baby was preterm and you haven't seen him/her yet, you should know that baby may not look exactly like what you expected. You may be bit alarmed at how tiny and fragile the baby seems. Preterm babies are naturally smaller than full-term babies; some may weigh less than two pounds.

Preterm babies are babies born before 37 weeks. For all practical purposes, we can divide these babies into 4 categories:

1) Late preterm 34+0 to 36+6 weeks.
2) Preterm 32+1 to 33+6 weeks and
3) Moderate Preterm babies born between 28+1 to 32 weeks.
4) Extreme Preterm babies born between 24 weeks to 28 weeks.

Viability is defined in India as 28 weeks. So for all practical purposes, we don't have proper statistics of any baby between 24 to 28 weeks ie., extreme preterm babies in India. Survival of babies and duration of stay for preterm babies depends on how preterm your baby is. Your neonatologist will be able to discuss these more in person with you. As a general rule,

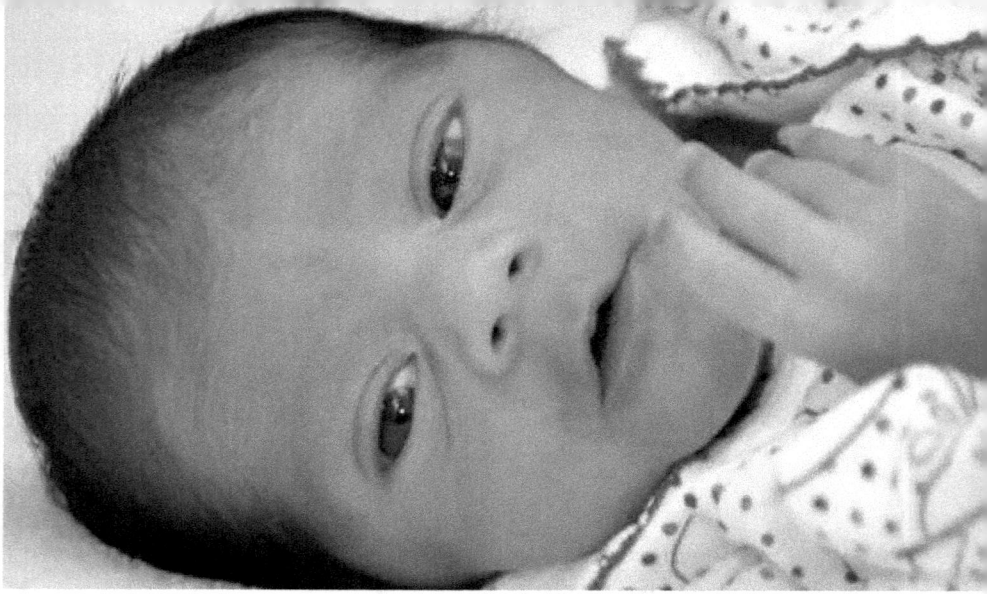

most babies go home after they reach 36 weeks of corrected weeks of gestation. At Cloudnine, we have had lot of babies born at less than 26 weeks and doing very well, please ask NICU staff to introduce the parents who have had premature babies in the past at Cloudnine, if you would like to speak to one such parent, so that you can understand first-hand what they went through.

A preterm baby is born with a thick, white coating covering its body, called vernix. After this is washed off, the baby's skin is red and wrinkled and may appear almost translucent in an extreme preterm situation. Tiny veins are visible below the skin's surface. Preterm babies of all ethnic groups have the same dusky-red skin color when they are born. Their natural skin color develops three to six weeks later.

During the last four weeks of pregnancy, a full-term baby gains a pound (200 gm) or so each week. The preterm baby misses out on this baby fat. The lack of fat filling out the skin folds gives a preterm baby a wrinkled appearance and makes his/her fingers, toes, and nose appear disproportionately.

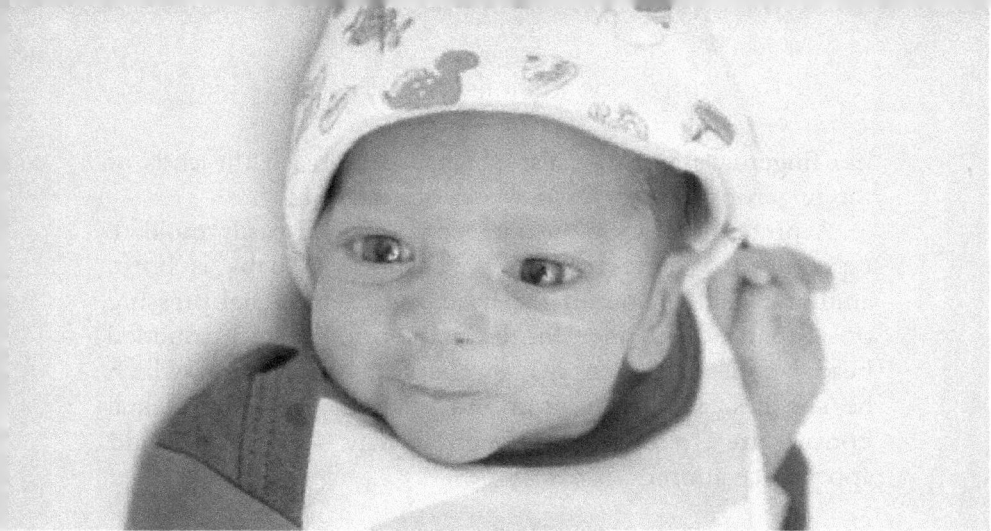

During the first few days of life, your baby will lose a few ounces. This is normal. It happens with full- term babies too. After that, he/she will probably gain up to an ounce (10-30 gm) or less each day. Babies' weight gain may fluctuate, losing an ounce or two some days, but still making good progress overall. Often, preterm babies take longer to regain their lost weight than full-term babies. The rate at which your baby gains weight helps the NICU staff tell how fast she/he is growing.

Your baby's facial features are well developed, except for his/her outer ears, which are still very soft and limp. They lie flat against his head and when they are folded over they do not spring back. As your baby continues to develop, his/her ears will form a firm layer of tissue that makes them look like those of a full-term baby. Since the 20th week of gestation, your baby's hair has been growing. By the time of preterm birth, it may cover the head. The hair will probably be very fine. Your baby may or may not have eyebrows and eyelashes. However, he/she have a light cover of hair on much of his/her body. This fetal hair, called lanugo may be quite heavy (especially around the shoulders), or it may merely be a light peachy fuzzy covering. This hair usually disappears in a few days or weeks. Even a very preterm baby has fingernails and toenails, which usually reach the ends of the fingertips or toes by 35 weeks of gestation.

A preterm baby's bones are very soft and easily molded, especially the bones of the skull. Before a baby is born, amniotic fluid surrounds the head and exerts equal pressure on all parts. But once the baby is born, the nice rounded head begins to flatten against the firm surfaces on which he/she lies. This elongation and flattening of the skull bones are temporary, though it may give an odd appearance at times.

Both preterm boys and girls have immature genitals, which may look unusual compared to those of a full-term baby. Your baby's sex organs may look larger than average. You can expect them to look more in proportion in a few weeks.

Like other babies, your baby will most likely stretch, yawn, and move his/her arms and legs. But because they lack muscle tone, they are usually very limp and flexible. In fact, some preterm babies like to sleep with their feet tucked up next to their heads. While this may look uncomfortable to you, it may be a position your baby enjoyed while still in your womb. You may also see your baby stiffen suddenly and then go limp. This is likely to happen because his/her nervous system isn't fully developed yet. Your baby does have a gripping reflex in the fingers, but this is too weak to maintain the grip when lifted by the hands. You may also see his/her arms and legs flail about with lots of jerks. This, too, is normal for preterm baby. As the baby matures, the movements will become smoother and more controlled.

Expect your baby to sleep most of the time as much as 15-22 hours a day at first. He/she may have a hard time being alert, but already some of the responses are like those of a full-term baby. You'll be able to see the baby cry, but you won't be able to hear, especially, if he/she's on a special breathing machine called a ventilator. This is because the tube from the machine sits in between their vocal cords.

You may wonder if your baby can see and hear. Right now, the baby hears better than he/she sees. The eyes may wander, and each eye may not even be looking in the same direction. Don't worry, sight will improve in time and our visiting Pediatric Ophthalmologist, will check your baby's eyes for Retinopathy of Prematurity (ROP), which is carried out for most preterm babies in NICU. Babies' hearing is a bit more advanced. You should talk to your baby. She/he's already know your voice, when they were in utero. It probably won't take him/her long to learn to respond to it. Talking to baby in a calm, soothing voice will comfort them. Babies can also sneeze, hiccup, smile, and may even suck their thumb, a skill acquired before birth.

Your gentle touches, being held and rocked, or being swaddled in a warm blanket may calm your baby. Most preterm babies like to be covered or firmly wrapped in a blanket. Our nurses at Cloudnine are trained to encourage parents to cuddle them at the earliest opportunity popularly we may use the term called KMC (for Kangaroo Mother Care) or KFC (for Kangaroo Father Care) this has shown to increase the bonding between the babies and their parents.

Even a very preterm baby can taste the difference between something sweet and something salty. Like most children, they tend to prefer the sweet. A full-term baby has a sense of smell so well developed that they can recognize their mother by scent alone. No one knows for sure what a preterm baby can smell, but some nurseries place an article of the mother's clothing in the baby's incubator with the hope that it will give a sense of his/her mother's comforting presence. Researchers have shown that babies who are exposed to mom's clothes are less agitated to compared to the ones who are not. For example, a handkerchief will allow

11

the baby to learn the natural scent of your skin. Avoid wearing perfumes that may seem harsh to the baby.

Even though your baby may be tiny and still in the NICU, he/she already is a special unique person with his/her own personality. You may even notice that she/he looks like his/her parents or siblings. It's just going to take some time for your baby to grow and develop. The best things you can do right now are taking care of yourself and spending time with your baby talking, touching, and giving the love your baby needs to grow strong.

YOUR THOUGHT PROCESS

During this stressful time, you may be experiencing a wide range of emotions. If you are like most parents of a preterm baby, the following may be passing through your mind.

- You may first feel shocked, and may be even anger.
- Why did this happen?
- What could I have done to prevent it?
- If I had only been more prepared for this

No matter how knowledgeable or well prepared you might have been, a preterm birth is still a uniquely challenging experience. As per Kubler Ross Model philosophy, any human being who goes through any emotional event which is not pleasant – will pass through 5 stages – Denial, Anger, Argument, Depression and Acceptance (DAADA). Initially you may feel denial, saying it cannot be happening to me, it must be a bad dream or something. At some point, you may also feel anger, guilt and depression. There may be times you want to argue with almost everyone & blame everyone - your spouse, the doctors, the world, and ultimately yourself. You may feel emotions like If I had only done this or hadn't done that. One word of advice - try not to torture yourself. Don't blame yourself for your baby's prematurity. Feelings of guilt and failure can interfere with your relationship with your baby. Talking with your NICU staff helps cope with these feelings.

In a maternity ward, surrounded by new moms and
their babies, you may feel alone and disappointed that
you missed the perfect birth experience and immediate joy
of motherhood that you envisioned while you were pregnant.
And, above all, you probably feel fear and anxiety. Will my
baby be okay? Will he/she survive? Try to remember, all
of these feelings are completely normal. They may change
on a day-to-day basis, or come in waves that make you feel
helpless and out of control. They are natural reactions that
most people in a crisis experience before they are ready to
accept their situation and adapt to it in a constructive way.
Let's now look at certain things you can do that may help you
stay motivated and positive.

Recognize that your feelings may be amplified by
postpartum depression, which affects some women in
varying degrees. Common postpartum feelings are tension,
anxiety and sadness. These emotions are probably because
of sudden hormonal changes after delivery. The fact that your
baby was preterm in no way changes this postpartum
chemistry. In fact, the preterm birth of your baby makes you
all the more vulnerable. Be patient with yourself and realize
what you're experiencing is, in fact, very normal.

Get all the rest you possibly can and eat well. Your body has just been through the exhausting experience of giving birth. Not getting enough rest, and not eating properly, will make it harder to regain the strength you will need to take care of yourself and your baby. In addition, depression and physical fatigue may also compound these feelings.

Talk! Talk to your spouse, your family, doctors, nurses, and friends. Keep communication open with each other and people who can give you comfort and strength. And cry if you want to, anytime, anyplace it's a necessary release.

Accept help from friends. Take friends or relatives up on their offers to care for your other children, if you have, drive you to the hospital, or run errands for you. Save your energy for visiting your baby.

Start a journal or diary. Keep a journal of your baby's progress, or write down your feelings, or both! Sometimes putting your thoughts on paper makes it easier to deal with them. Read! Reading everything you can about your baby's conditions or preterm delivery will give you a better understanding of the current situation. The feelings of knowing and understanding will give you a better feeling of control.

Look at your baby's picture. Remember the old saying, A picture is worth a thousand words? In this case, it could be a thousand smiles. Taking pictures of your baby will help you feel closer to your baby even when you can't be with him/her. Also, continue to take pictures on a regular basis. You may not recognize your baby's progress until you actually see it in a photo.

Join a support group, if you have one. At Cloudnine, we can certainly introduce you to the other mothers who have had preterm babies before at your request. Sharing your thoughts and feelings with others who have been, or currently are, in your situation is often a great form of comfort and stress release. It's also a great place to learn from and be motivated by others who have been through it.

VISITING YOUR BABY

As your baby grows stronger in the NICU, there is a special job to be done that only you can do - give plenty of loving attention to your baby. Your love and contact are just as critical to your baby's wellbeing as the food, warmth, and oxygen he/she needs to survive. The NICU staff recognizes this and invites you to visit your baby as often as possible. At Cloudnine, we encourage parents to visit their baby every day.

When you visit your baby for the first time, he/she may look different than what you expected or remember. You may be shocked at how small and helpless he/she may seem. You may feel an overwhelming need to protect him/her. You may even feel like crying. It's okay. Cry if you need to. Everyone caring for your baby understand that. They help parents just like you every day.

You may see the medical staff and a lot of equipment that are unfamiliar. Though some of the equipment may seem intimidating or frightening at first, each piece is very important to take care of your baby. In the section of this book, entitled "An Introduction to the Equipment in the NICU", we'll help you get familiar with some of the

17

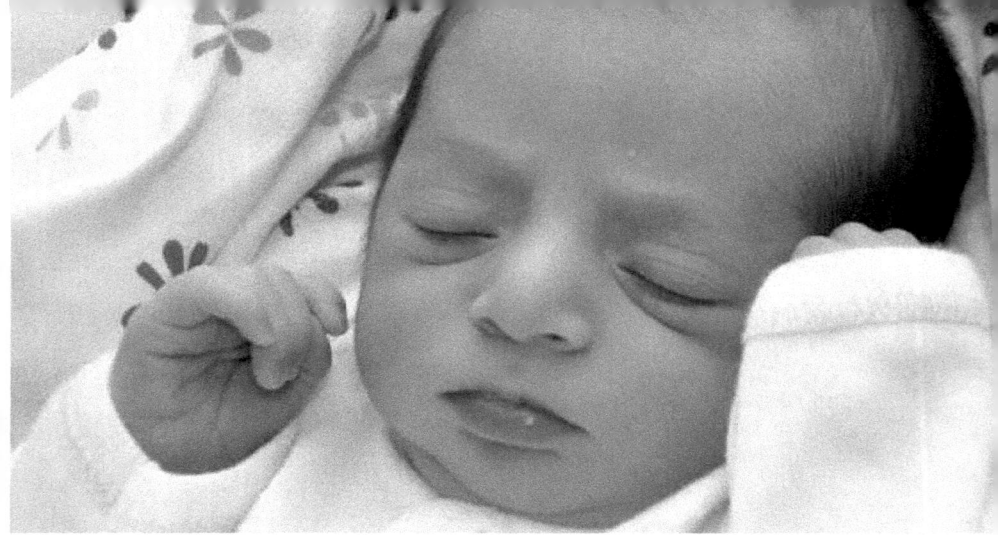

equipment you may see. In addition, on your first visit, your doctor/nurse will explain the equipment used for your baby. Your NICU staff wants you to be informed and feel as comfortable as possible. All these equipment are used to monitor various functions of the baby to ensure that anything not going well is picked up immediately.

Since the NICU is a busy place, you'll need to ask about the rules and visiting guidelines before you visit. Your NICU staff can tell you the best times to visit your baby. Visits to your baby may also be more enjoyable if they coincide with his/her natural periods of alertness, though as a mother you can visit your baby anytime of the day or night. A very tiny or sick baby may have very few periods of alertness. The interactions you can have may be limited at first. As your baby grows, the alert periods will lengthen and the tolerance for stimulation will increase. Most parents may want to target feeding times because the baby is most likely to be alert and begin to associate feeding time with Mom.

Remember, your preterm baby, like the rest of us, may have good and bad days. Your baby may not be able to tolerate too much stimulation at one time. No two preterm babies are alike. One may love to be rocked for hours, while another is overwhelmed by the slightest touch. Don't worry, your NICU staff will be there to guide you at every stage.

During your visits, your NICU nurses may ask you to wear a gown and wash your hands in a special way to prevent germs from being spread to your baby. They may also ask you to wear a mask over your mouth and nose, if you seem to have a cold or cough to ensure your baby doesn't get infected.

If your baby is going to be in the NICU for a long time (depending on how preterm your baby is) and if you have other children at home wanting to see their new sibling, talk with your NICU staff about arranging visits. In Cloudnine your baby may be hooked on to a small tiny camera – with which you may see your baby 24/7 on your smartphone. The NICU staff will do everything possible to involve your entire family in your baby's care, with certain limitations to reduce the chances of infection in the NICU. You may also encourage your older children to color or draw a picture for the baby to be left at the nursery. Allowing them to bring a gift may help them feel more in touch with the baby until he/she comes home.

The time your baby is in the NICU may be a trying, stressful time for your entire family. Just remember, it won't last forever. Your baby is growing stronger every day. Visit your baby as often as possible. Your love is the best medicine your baby can receive.

20

UNDERSTANDING THE NICU

The letters NICU stand for Neonatal Intensive Care Unit. This is the special place where specially trained doctors and nurses are giving your baby round-the-clock care. This kind of special care is too involved to provide in a standard newborn nursery. Not all hospitals have NICUs, so your baby may have been transferred here from the facility where he/she was born. The goal of the NICU staff is the same as yours - to help baby grow and become healthy enough to go home with you where he/she belongs.

At first the NICU may seem like a stark, bleak, and very noisy place filled with tubes, wires, dials, bright lights, and alarms. Most of the equipment attached to the babies have a built-in-alarm system. Anytime the equipment's monitoring systems sense a change, an alarm sounds to alert the staff. These alarms do not always mean something is wrong with the baby, but they may require a response from the staff. Don't let the sound of the NICU scare you. The staff watch these machines closely and is always prepared to take care of any problem that may occur.

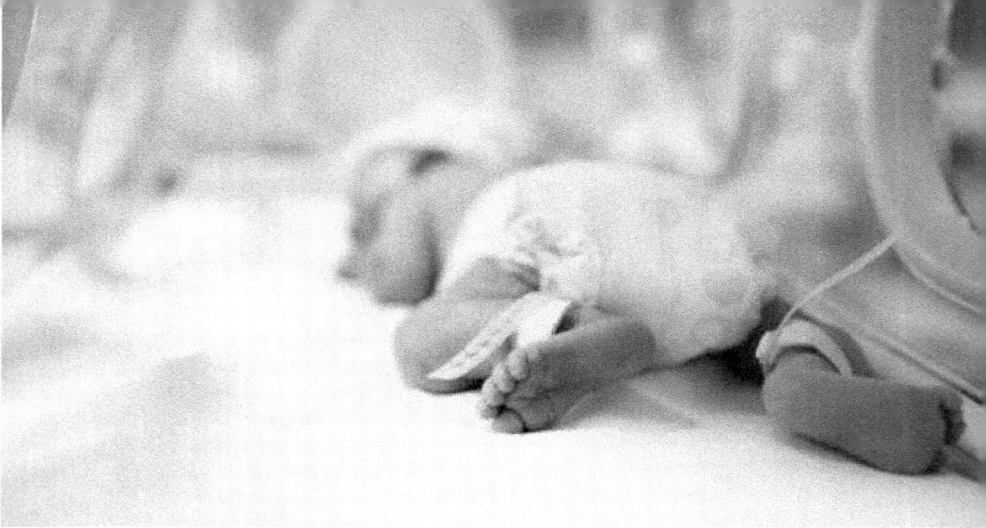

Sometimes babies need to stay in the NICU because of something that occurred during birth or because some organ or system isn't functioning the way it should. But frequently, babies are placed in the NICU simply because they were born too soon (prematurely).

To help you become familiar with the people caring for your baby, we have listed the titles and descriptions of your NICU staff below. Use this as a general guideline. Your hospital may have fewer or more members on their NICU staff.

Neonatologist: A pediatrician (children's doctor) with advanced training in the area of intensive care of newborn medicine. You will find that the neonatologist in charge of the NICU unit keeps changing. These doctors work on a rotating basis to give your baby the best care possible. The neonatologist in charge is called the neonatologist on-call .

Fellow: A fully trained and experienced pediatric (children's) doctor who is training to become a neonatologist.

Registrar: A medical doctor specialized in pediatrics - he/she is actively involved in your baby's care and is a good resource for information.

Neonatal Nurse Practitioner: A nurse who has completed an advanced educational program in neonatology and works under the direction of the neonatologist. Most of these nurses have more than 2 decades of experience, sometimes they are a good source of information & also for counselling.

NICU Nurses: Your baby will have one or more nurses assigned to each shift. Shifts may vary between eight and twelve hours. These nurses are specially trained to care for the babies.

Primary Nurse: The primary nurse plans your baby's nursing care. She is responsible for getting to know you and your baby, and any special needs you may have.

Physiotherapists: In the NICU, physiotherapists are important members of the health care team. Physiotherapists are specially trained to care for babies with muscle problems or breathing difficulties.

Other Caregivers: In addition to the above mentioned team, depending on your baby's needs, the care of other specialized doctors may also be required. They will be introduced to you as and when, if necessary for your baby's care like Paediatric Ophthalmologists, Paediatric Cardiologists and even Neonatal/Pediatric Surgeons.

While this may seem like a lot of information to process, you will soon learn and become comfortable. The NICU staff are working for you and your baby and are there to help you in any way they can.

SPECIAL CONDITIONS OF PREMATURITY

In a medical field as rapidly evolving and improving as neonatology, there are bound to be variations from hospital to hospital in terminology, technology, and treatments. Your doctor may use slightly different terms to describe some of the medical conditions discussed here. New methods to treat the potential medical problems of the preterm baby are constantly evolving. The purpose of this section is to introduce you to some potential medical problems of preterm babies and some of the methods involved for treating and correcting the problems. We hope that with this basic information you will be better able to discuss the specifics of your baby's care with your neonatologist and NICU staff.

Need for Warmth

From the time of conception, your baby was nurtured inside the warmth of your body. At birth, they emerged wet into a cold world where they suddenly need to regulate their own body temperature. It is almost like going from India to Antarctica! A full-term baby who gains a pound of fat a week during the last weeks before birth is relatively well insulated. A preterm baby, however, is very vulnerable to

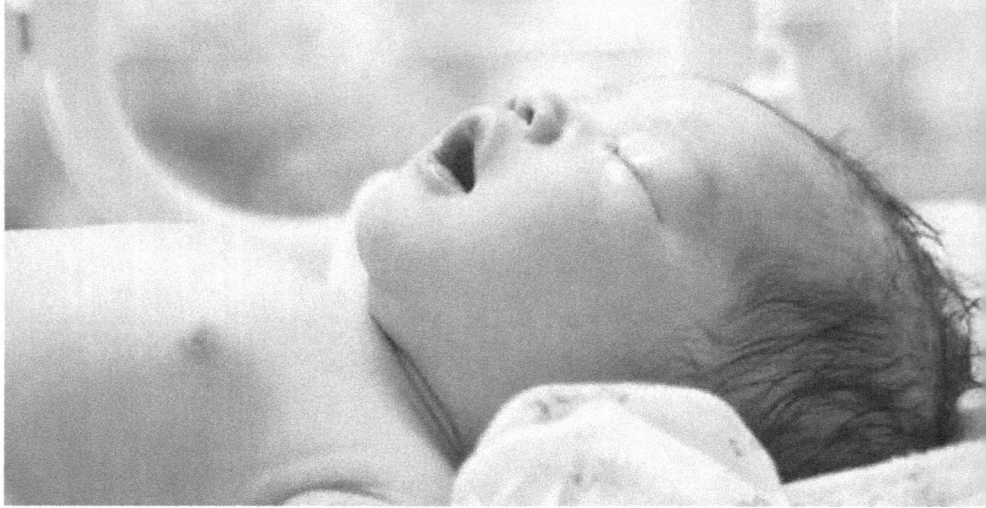

cold. A 1500 grams baby may lose five times the amount of heat per unit of body weight as an adult does.

A preterm baby, especially a baby with breathing problems, is poorly supplied with calories and oxygen fuels a baby needs to regulate heat in the body. Because of the potential dangers, the main objective of your NICU staff is to keep your baby warm, but not too warm. Your baby's temperature must be carefully controlled in an incubator or warmer. A tiny device that acts as a thermometer is taped to your baby's stomach. It constantly senses your baby's temperature and regulates the temperature of the environment. It will increase the warmth when your baby gets too cold and decrease it when he is too warm. Your baby's axillary (under the arm) temperature will be checked frequently as well.

The goal is to keep your baby's body temperature as close to normal as possible, i.e. 98.6 F (37.0 C). This is also the temperature at which they conserve the most oxygen and calories, and gain the most weight.

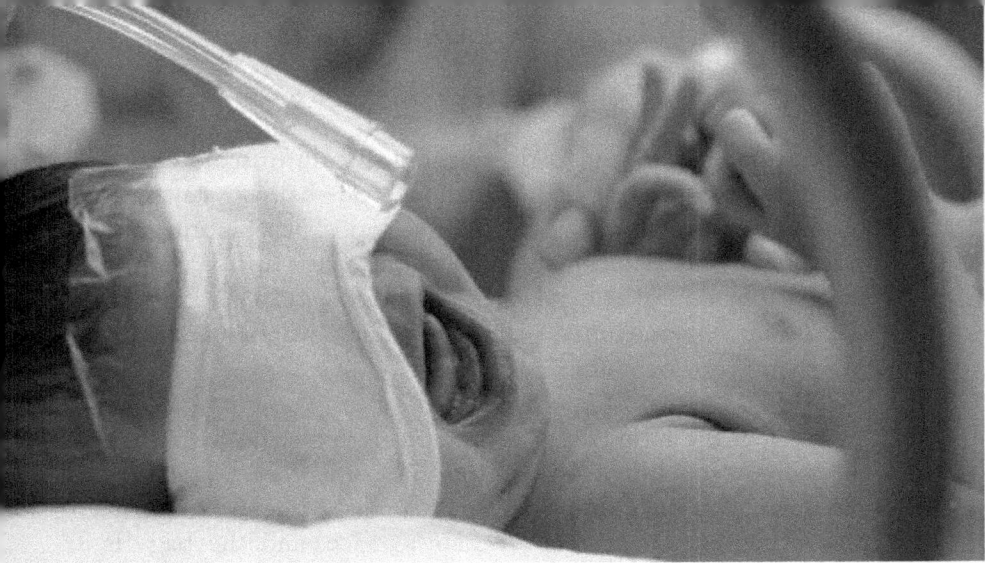

Breathing

It's very common for preterm babies to have breathing problem. The severity of the problem may depend on how prematurely your baby was born. A preterm baby's lungs aren't as fully developed and ready to breathe as a full-term baby's. Let us now look at some common problems associated with breathing.

Apnea & Bradycardia

Apnea is the term used to describe the times a baby stops breathing. Apnea is very common among preterm babies in the early weeks of life. Apnea is often accompanied by Bradycardia - a lower-than-normal heart rate. For a tiny baby this means the heart is beating lesser than 100 times a minute. This is considered low for a baby, even though an adult heart rate is usually much lower.

In the NICU, your baby will be closely watched for signs of Apnea and Bradycardia with the help of electronic monitoring. Small adhesive monitoring pads or sensors are placed on the baby's skin to detect chest movements as they breathe, and to pick up the impulses of their heartbeat.

Wires attached to the pads transmit the information to a machine next to your baby's bed. If your baby's vital signs become abnormal, an alarm will sound. These monitoring machines only detect your baby's heartbeat and breathing rates - they do not control them in any way. In addition to the monitoring machines, your NICU nurse will be personally observing your baby for any changes.

Most of the time breathing can be started again by patting the baby or touching/stroking the soles of its feet. Sometimes the nurse may have to do bagging - a mask attached to a soft plastic bag is placed on the baby's face, and the bag is squeezed many times to push air into the lungs and trigger the breathing cycle.

Respiratory Distress Syndrome (RDS)

RDS is a breathing disorder found in preterm babies. It is caused by the baby's inability to produce surfactant. This is the fatty substance that coats the alveoli, the tiny air sacs in the lungs, and keeps them from collapsing.

An unborn baby's lung tissue begins making small amounts of surfactant in the early weeks of pregnancy, but most babies aren't producing enough surfactant for proper breathing until the 34th week of gestation. However, babies do vary greatly in their rates of lung development. Some preterm babies have enough surfactant - to keep their lungs open, breathe without difficulty - while some do not. The more preterm a baby is, the greater the risk of developing RDS.

RDS treatment is nothing but helping the baby with the breathing process. Some babies may be given surfactant - a substance to help mature the lungs. The baby may be given oxygen and a variety of other medical treatments to aid breathing and circulation until he/she is able to produce surfactant and cure itself. After the first three or four days, depending on how prematurely the baby was born, your baby's lungs may begin to produce enough surfactant for him/her to breathe normally.

Pulmonary Interstitial Emphysema (PIE) and Pneumothorax (new'-moh-thor'ax)

When it is necessary for your baby to be on a ventilator, the pressure may occasionally cause air to leak from their lungs. Tiny air bubbles may be forced out of the alveoli and in between layers of lungs tissue. This condition, called pulmonary interstitial emphysema (PIE), usually subsides as the baby's respiratory problems improve and ventilator pressure to the lungs is reduced. It is much rarer nowadays.

Sometimes a tear can occur in the membrane that covers the baby's lungs, or one or more of the alveoli in his/her lungs can burst. This causes air to leak into the surrounding chest spaces and can cause the lung to collapse. This is called pneumothorax. To treat this problem, a small plastic tube may be placed in the chest (under local anesthesia) to suck out the air between the lung and the chest wall. This allows the lung to re-inflate. The suction continues for a few days until the lung heals. The chest tube is then removed.

Umbilical Catheter (UAC & UVC)

The umbilical catheter is inserted through the end of a baby's umbilical cord (belly button) and is threaded through the umbilical artery into the aorta, the main artery supplying the body with oxygenated blood (called UAC Umbilical Arterial Catheter) and through the umbilical vein into the inferior vena cava, the main vein returning the blood from lower half of the body to the heart (called UVC Umbilical Venous Catheter). While this sounds painful, it really isn't. There are no nerve endings in your baby's belly button where the catheter (tiny tube) is inserted.

The catheter is a convenient, painless way for the NICU staff to draw blood frequently without having to re-stick your baby with a needle every time. It also allows fluids, nutrients, blood and medications to be easily given to your baby. A device attached to the catheter also constantly monitors your baby's blood pressure. The catheter will be removed when it is no longer necessary.

IV Pump/Superficial IV/Syringe pump IV

An IV pump is a machine attached to a pole placed near your baby's bed. IV stands for intravenous, which means into the veins. To start an IV on your baby, a cannula is inserted into a superficial vein (one that is close to the skins surface), with a very small intravenous cannula. If the IV is in the arm or leg, the limb may be splinted with a spatula and covered with a piece of gauze so that the baby cant dislodge the cannula, which is plastic and does not hurt the baby.

Nutrients, medication and blood can be given through the superficial IV, but blood cannot be withdrawn because the superficial veins are too fragile. If your baby needs frequent blood samplings then he/she may need to have two IV lines or the umbilical catheter for drawing blood and a superficial IV for feeding and medications.

AN INTRODUCTION TO THE EQUIPMENT IN NICU

This section is designed to give you a general understanding of some of the equipments you may see in the NICU.

Warmer

A warmer is a bed designed to try & keep your baby at the right temperature. It is similar to an incubator in its function, but is not enclosed like a box. It is more like a bed with warmth being provided to your baby from a heat source above the bed. However, your baby will have a small device, which acts like a thermometer, taped to his body. The thermometer signals heat to be increased or decreased as per your baby's needs.

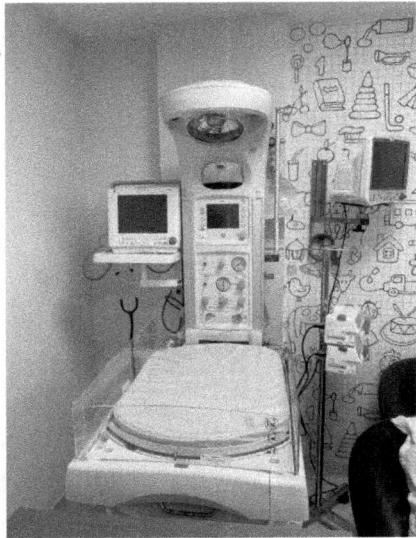

Incubator

An incubator is a heated plastic enclosure that you can see through. It provides a controlled temperature & humid environment which helps to keep your baby warm, lessens the water loss through skin and at the correct temperature. As your baby's body varies in temperature, heat is increased or decreased accordingly.

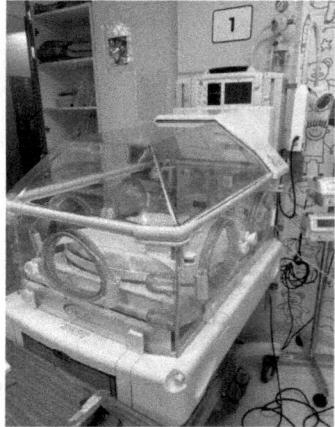

In most Cloudnine Hospitals we have specialized equipment from GE called Giraffe which is like an artificial womb - it is a hybrid of both warmer and incubator and the nurses will familiarize you with this, if required. It is more like the Rolls Royce of incubators!

Multipara Monitor

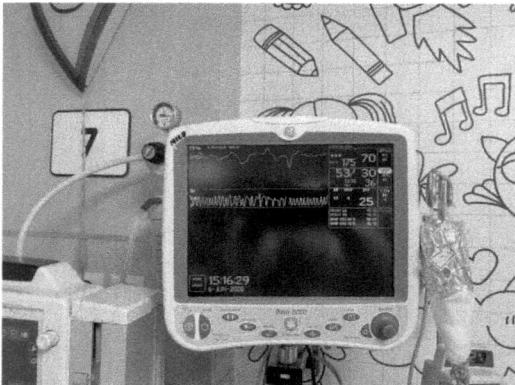

A multipara monitor is an equipment used to monitor your baby's heart rate, breathing, oxygen saturation, temperature and blood pressure. Small adhesive monitoring pads, referred to as electrodes or patches, are placed on a baby's skin to detect chest movements as they breathe and to pick up the impulses of their heartbeat. Wires attached to the pads transmit this information to the monitor next to the baby's bed. If the baby's vital signs become abnormal, an alarm will sound which alerts the NICU staff.

Oxygen Hood

An oxygen hood is used for babies who can breathe on their own, but still need extra oxygen. Oxygen can be piped directly into the baby's incubator, but if high or precisely measured doses of oxygen are required, a plastic box or dome, called an oxygen hood, is placed over the baby's head, through which warm and moist oxygenated air flows into the hood. An oxygen analyzer, placed beside the baby's head, double-checks the amount of oxygen he/she is receiving.

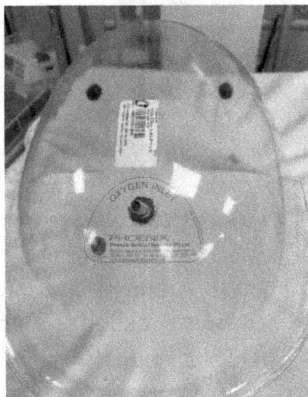

Oxygen Mask

An oxygen mask is a mask placed over the baby's nose and mouth. Oxygen flows through a tube and into the mask at a constant rate. It may be used during CPAP (explained below) instead of nasal prongs or an endo-tracheal tube, or at other times when increased oxygen is necessary.

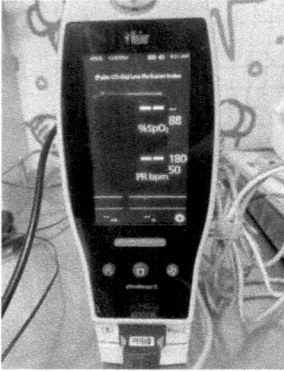

Pulse Oximeter

A pulse oximeter is a device that non-invasively monitors and determines a baby's arterial blood oxygen saturation and pulse.

Nasal Prongs

Nasal prongs are used to help your baby breathe in a treatment called Continuous Positive Airway Pressure (CPAP) or High Flow Nasal Cannula (HFNC). Through this procedure, pressurized air is delivered to your baby's lungs through small tubes placed inside your baby's nostrils. These tubes provide a steady stream of oxygen. The oxygen may also be delivered for CPAP through a facemask or an endo-tracheal tube at times.

Endo-tracheal Tube

An endo-tracheal tube is a very small, slender tube which is passed through a baby's nose or mouth, past the vocal cords (voice box) and down into the trachea (windpipe). This process may also be referred to as intubation. The tube is attached to a machine (a ventilator) that pumps air & oxygen into the lungs, under controlled pressure & volume,

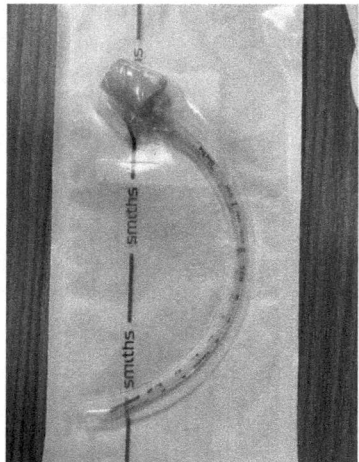

to assist in breathing.

Ventilator

A baby who is having frequent spells of apnea, or is too weak to breathe well on its own is intubated and the endotracheal tube is attached to a ventilator. This machine does the breathing for the baby, till the baby can breathe on its own.

The ventilator performs several functions. It delivers a measured amount of oxygen to the baby's lungs with each breath and also provides constant pressure and/or volume to keep the lungs open. At regular intervals the machine inhales for the baby by pushing in additional air at a higher pressure. The oxygen content of the air, the pressure, and the number of breaths per minute the baby needs, can all be adjusted, as required from time to time. The NICU staff determine the baby's needs by observing the baby and by measuring the oxygen, carbon dioxide, and acid levels in the baby's bloodstream through blood gases (ABG).

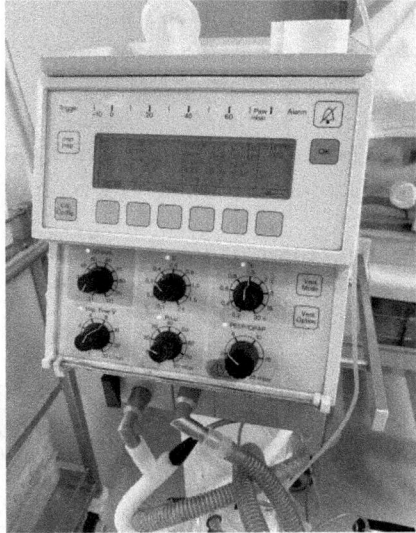

Suction Catheter

A baby with breathing problems cannot cough up the mucus that accumulates in the lungs. These secretions must be removed for them by the process called suctioning. These processes include a variety of methods to loosen the mucus. Once the mucus has been loosened, the baby's endo-tracheal tube is detached from the ventilator. A suctioning tube (or catheter) is quickly inserted through the endo-tracheal tube and into the baby's trachea to vacuum up any secretions.

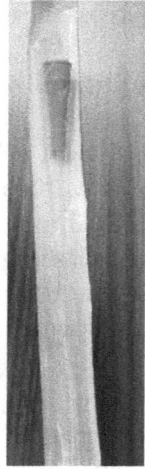

Bili-blankets

Babies with high jaundice are treated by a process called phototherapy. This is done by placing your baby under

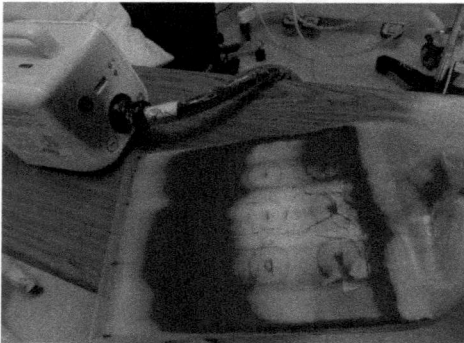

special bright light called bililights or LED lights. These fluorescent lights are placed over your baby's incubator. A mask or eye patch will be placed over your baby's eyes to assure their comfort and prevent any potential damage from the lights, just like sun-glasses. Or, your baby may be wearing a bili-blanket, which eliminates the need to cover the baby's eyes during therapy.

The blue light waves from the LED or bililights change the molecular structure of the bilirubin, which allows it to be transported to the liver, detoxified (broken down) and excreted from your baby's body. If your baby is under phototherapy, he/she will be without clothing, so that as much skin as possible can be exposed to the light.

While undergoing phototherapy, your baby's bowel movements may be frequent, loose and maybe even greenish in color. Babies also tend to sleep a lot while being treated for jaundice, waking only for feedings. Phototherapy will be continued, usually one to three days, until the bilirubin level in your baby's blood is reduced to a normal range.

JAUNDICE IN NEWBORNS

Jaundice in newborn babies, especially preterm babies is normal and is not serious most of the times.

What is jaundice?

Jaundice is a yellow color of your baby's skin. The whites of your baby's eyes may be yellow. This is due to excess amount of a pigment called BILIRUBIN.

The bilirubin comes from the breakdown of red blood cells. This type of jaundice starts when baby is 2 or 3 days old. It goes away by the time your baby is 2 to 3 weeks old. This happens in about half of all babies and is not harmful. If the jaundice appears on the very first day, it is not normal and your Paediatrician will discuss more about it. Jaundice progresses from head to toes. It regresses from below upwards; whites of the eyes may remain yellow longer, for up to 2 to 3 weeks.

This could happen for any of these reasons and almost ALL preterm babies get jaundice in the first week of life.

Normal Jaundice: There are several reasons for this:

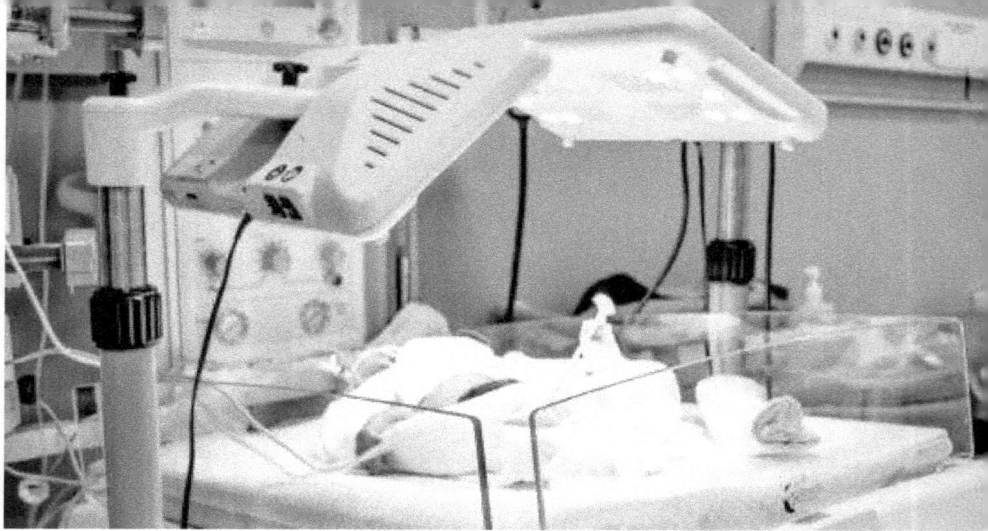

- The baby's liver just isn't ready to get rid of the yellow pigment called bilirubin on its own.
- During birth, babies receive more blood from the placenta than they can handle immediately.
- Some babies can be bruised at birth - bruises produce more bilirubin.
- The gut motility in the first few days sometimes isn't that good. So babies take some time before they can 'excrete' bilirubin in the stools.

Rh or ABO problems: Jaundice can happen if mother and baby have different blood groups or types. There are two different types of blood group incompatibility that can cause jaundice. When the mother's blood group is O positive and the baby's group is A,B or AB positive; or when the mother's blood type is negative and the baby's type is positive, jaundice can occur in the baby.

At Cloudnine, we routinely check every baby's blood group – so we will know about this, if this is the case. This type of jaundice most often starts from the first day of life. Please ask your Paediatrician for further information.

Your baby can also get jaundice by:
  - Being born too early or preterm

- Getting bruises from the birth
- Infection and diseases

How is jaundice treated?

Most babies with jaundice may not require any treatment, but preterm babies generally have higher chance of requiring treatment.

When your baby looks more jaundiced, a blood test is done again to check the level of bilirubin and if required to reduce the level of jaundice – the baby is to exposed to light, a process called phototherapy. We have specialized lights called "biliblanket & LED lights" – with which we treat the babies and with these new technologies – the speed at which bilirubin comes to normal levels is much faster and also the baby stays within the incubator rather than being taken out of it unlike in most hospitals. These are harmless and painless treatment. The lights change the bilirubin, so that the kidneys can get rid of it rather than the liver, which can be immature in newborn babies more so in preterm babies. The baby's eyes are covered to protect them from the bright light, just like you wear sunglasses when you go out in the bright sun. Your baby may develop skin rashes or pass loose, greenish bowel movements. If these were to happen, it is temporary and should stop when the phototherapy is discontinued. Phototherapy is safe, but is used only when needed.

Breast Milk Jaundice (BMJ): it is normal for breastfeeding babies to have jaundice lasting bit longer. It usually occurs at 10 -21 days of age, and can last for 2 -3 months. As long as baby is gaining weight, passing lots of clear yellow urine and yellow or green stools and having bowel movements, there is no need to be worried. It is not harmful. Do no stop breastfeeding or expressing breast milk. BMJ is a sort of diagnosis of exclusion – in Cloudnine all babies are tested for "newborn screening disorders" – which sort of rules out majority of the causes. If the baby is active, passing yellow stools – most of the time, nothing else need to be done. If these newborn screening tests have not been done, then the baby needs to be subjected to a few tests to ensure – there is no other reason for the same.

TESTS AND EXAMS

As soon as your baby is taken to the NICU, the staff may immediately begin a series of procedures, tests and exams to determine what treatment is necessary. This is done quickly so that the staff can start the necessary treatments without delay. The tests will continue throughout your baby's stay in the NICU to monitor the progress and react to any changes as necessary.

Our NICU staff will be communicating these with you on a constant basis and advising you of tests and procedures. No major test, procedures or operations will be performed without your knowledge and approval, **unless it is an emergency.** Most of the tests your baby will receive initially are routine. These include checking heart rate, blood sugar, blood pressure and temperature. In addition, your baby will be weighed and have blood tests done to check infection and next day ultrasound imaging studies will be done to ensure there is no bleeding in the brain and sometimes to check blood pressure in the lungs called pulmonary hypertension.

Weighing

Weighing is a very simple and much-needed procedure. Weight gain is very important and is almost a sure sign of progress for preterm babies. To make sure your baby is gaining weight, the nurses will measure and record the exact amounts of fluid and breast milk or formula that the baby receives. Baby's bowel movements will also be monitored and their output recorded. In the NICU, babies' weights are measured in grams.

Blood Tests

Your baby will undergo blood tests while staying in the NICU. Blood tests can tell a lot about their overall condition as well as alert the doctors to any potential or actual problems. Sometimes babies who don't have enough red blood cells, or have a serious blood disease or disorder, may require a blood transfusion. Frequent blood tests enable doctors to quickly react to any changes or problems your baby may experience.

One test your baby may have is a blood gases check. A seriously ill baby has blood gases checked several times each day. A baby in a more stable condition may be tested once or twice a day. These tests are very important. They indicate how well the gases, i.e. oxygen and carbon dioxide, are being exchanged between the lungs and the bloodstream. In addition to it, if your baby is ill, they will show the effect the baby's illness is having on the acid content of his/her blood. These tests are repeated often because changes in a baby's blood chemistry can occur rapidly.

Samples of blood to be tested for oxygen, carbon dioxide and acid may be taken from the baby's arteries, since it is the arterial blood that supplies the body tissue with oxygen. Arterial blood can be withdrawn from the aorta through the umbilical artery catheter, or from arteries in the baby's wrist, foot or scalp. If a drop or two of blood is needed, the blood may be taken by pricking the baby's heel.

Imaging Studies

Imaging simply means making pictures of organs and other structures inside your baby's body. There are several common types of imaging your baby may need while in the NICU. These procedures are necessary to allow your doctor to track your baby's progress and be aware of any special conditions.

X-rays

An x-ray is the most common type of imaging exam. If your baby has breathing problems, he/she may be x-rayed as often as several times a day. This is done to evaluate the condition of his/her lungs and other organs, and to check the positions of tubes or catheter inside her body,

When you were pregnant, you were probably warned against the dangers of x-rays. With this in mind, the thought of your baby being x-rayed frequently may make you worried or concerned about any negative effect an x-ray could have on your baby. This is a valid concern on your part, but there's absolutely no reason to worry. Because the x-ray machines used for babies have very low doses of radiation which, experts agree are too low to cause any harm to your baby, now or in the future. The NICU staff may also leave the area while your baby is being x-rayed. This is precaution they take since even small amounts of scatter radiation may become significant to a person who is exposed all day, every day, for many years.

Ultrasound

An ultrasound picture is like an x-ray, except that it is composed of sound waves (and has no radiation) aimed at organs in the body. The sound waves send back different types of echoes that indicate the density of the tissue they are examining. Ultrasound scans may be performed at your baby's bedside. They are simple, painless procedures that require no sedation of your baby. They have no side effects.

CT Scans and MRI Pictures

The term CT or CAT Scan stands for Computerized Axial Tomography scan and MRI stands for Magnetic Resonance Imaging. These two are advanced types of imaging that performed when doctors need to know more than they can learn from x-rays or ultrasound. They are frequently used to examine your baby's brain. They work as a sort of combination of an x-ray machine and a computer. They aim a very narrow beam of radiation (CT) or magnetic waves (MRI) at a specific layer of body tissue and produce a horizontal or cross-sectional picture. Your baby will have to be taken to the x-ray department because the machines are much too large to move. Your baby may also need to be sedated because the baby must be completely still during the scans. These scans are also painless procedures for your baby.

Birth details / Obstetric discharge summary

Name of the Baby :---------

Name of the Hospital :   Branch: City:

Date of Birth: -----   Time of birth: ------

Obstetrician's Name: ----------

Maternal information

Mother's Name:------

Blood group:----------   Anti D given: Yes / No...............

Pregnancy complications:-----------

Delivery: Vaginal delivery / vacuum extraction / forceps / elective LSCS / non-elective LSCS

Partner present at birth: Yes / No...----------

Intra / Post partum complications:----------

Neonatal information

Estimated gestation: ---- weeks   Apgar: 1 minute:---------- 5 minutes:-----

Abnormalities noted at birth and problems requiring treatment:---------------

Birth weight (kg):---- Birth length(cm)------- Birth head cir. (cm):-------

Newborn blood tests:

Blood group:----- Guthrie:---- date:--- other(specify):------ date:-------
Vitamin K given: Injection Y/ N ----   Oral: 1st dose: -------- 2nd dose:------- 3rd dose:----

Feeding at discharge: Breast / EBM / Formula:----------
Difficulties with feeding:--------

Date of discharge:------- Discharge weigh (kg):---------
H.C (cm):--------

Signature:-------- Designation:----------- Date:------------

Newborn Screening test for Biochemical Disorders

Newborn Screening tests (popularly called in some countries as Guthrie test or a heal prick test) is test done on all babies in most developed countries routinely. In India, its awareness is not much and hence not widely known. Just like how we examine your baby for any physical abnormality, newborn screening test examines your baby for any "biochemical abnormality" ex: underactive thyroid (hypothyroidism) which if not tested, may not be obvious till the baby becomes mentally retarded later. The technology exists to test nearly 50 such diseases with one drop of blood on a filter paper and this is done routinely for all babies especially premature babies – but babies have to have had feeds before this test is done. Hence sometimes we may do this test twice in premature babies – once before any blood transfusion is given and if they baby has not been fed by that time, will repeat 6 weeks after the last blood transfusion so that we get accurate results. The 50 odd disorders we test are grouped under 9 disease headings as below:

Disease	Date done	Pass	Refer	Repeat Test
Congenital Hypothyroidism				
G6PD Deficiency				
Galactosaemia				
Cystic Fibrosis				
Amino Acid Disorders				
Fatty Acid Oxidation Defects				
Congenital Adrenal Hyperplasia				
Biotinidase Deficiency				
Haemoglobinopathies				
Optional: Cord blood Vitamin D levels				
Cord blood DHA levels				

Preterm babies are at risk of deafness both because of prematurity itself and also due to various other reasons including some life saving drugs used to treat them. Hence all babies are tested for hearing with the hearing screening methods before discharge to ensure adequate speech development. This is a routine test and nothing to be worried about and it is a painless test.

Newborn Hearing Screening test by AABR Method

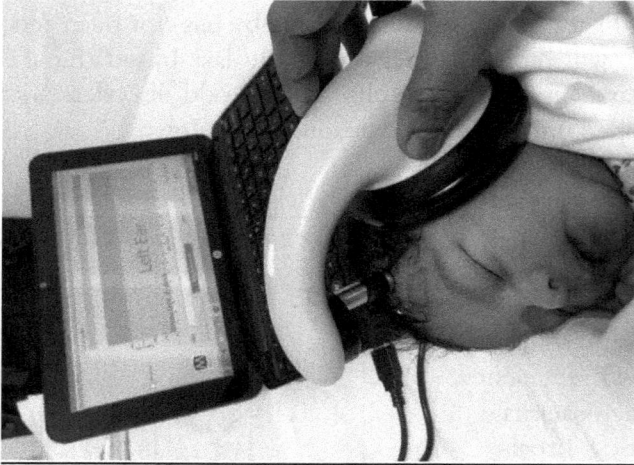

Left Ear Testing

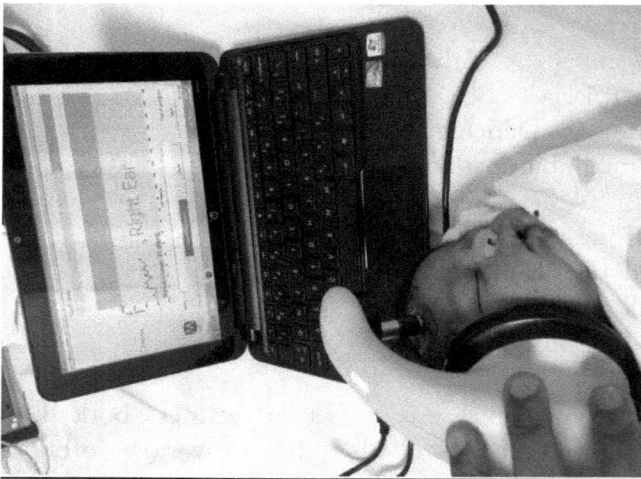

Right Ear Testing

Newborn hearing test	Date	Pass	Refer	Test
			R: L:	

Newborn Screening test for Critical Cyanotic Congenital Heart Diseases

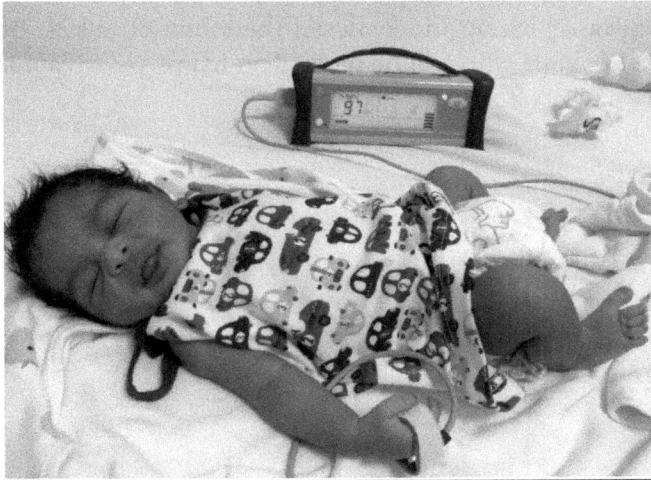

CCCHD Screening

The risk of a baby being born with congenital heart disease is 1:800, which is very common. There is a subgroup of heart diseases in newborn babies called Critical Cyanotic Heart Diseases, which if diagnosed early have a better chance of the baby surviving. Hence, all babies are screened for this by checking oxygen saturation levels in all 4 limbs. Generally we do this test within the first few days of life. This is again a painless test.

SpO2 test for CCHD detection @ birth	Date	Pass	Refer	Test
RUL RLL LUL LLL			R: L:	

If you need any further information on any of the above tests, please pick up the leaflet in the lobby or talk to one of the NICU staff who will be more than happy to explain about them.

FEEDINGS

Before your baby was born, he/she received a steady flow of carefully selected, predigested nutrients that crossed the placenta from your body into his/her through umbilical vessels and the placenta. In other words, you were the perfect food source. Because he/she was born too early, your baby was removed from that food source before being ready to eat and digest food on his/her own. Good nutrition may never be more important to your baby than it is right now.

Nutrition is a very complex science. Your baby's nutritional needs are also complex and very different than those of an adult. You may already know that your baby needs protein, carbohydrates vitamins, and minerals, but you might be surprised to learn about the needs for fat. Breast milk, the ideal food source for nearly all babies, is about 50% fat. Fat provides highly concentrated energy for growth and tissue-building material for the brain, eyes, and central nervous system.

Health care professionals recommend feeding babies breast milk. Even though breast milk fills unique needs for your baby, sometimes it needs to be fortified to provide the best growth possible. If you are unable to breastfeed, or choose not to do so, donor breast milk can be considered as an alternative or a special infant formula, such as Pre-Nan or Neo-Sure may be used. Premature formula provides excellent nutrition for your baby. It provides a balance of nutrients especially designed to meet the special nutrition needs of the preterm babies, but may not be as good as breast milk.

Don't be alarmed if your baby is too weak or too ill to breastfeed or bottle-feed while he/she is in the NICU. There are other ways to provide the babies with the nutrition they need. In this section, we will discuss some of those ways, along with breastfeeding, bottle-feeding and tips for feeding your baby.

Types of Feedings

IV Feedings

A baby with breathing problems or an extremely premature baby cannot be given anything by mouth at first. Their immature digestive tract must slowly and cautiously be introduced to its new role in providing nourishment. Also if a baby is too sick or stressed, he/she may have poor circulation in the digestive tract. This is because the body reacts to stress by temporarily shunting blood to the most critical organs needed to survive the heart, brain, kidneys and lungs, instead of those such as the stomach and intestines. Because a premature baby may be using most of his/her energy just to breathe at first, it is unlikely that anything given by mouth would be properly digested. Therefore, many premature babies receive their first feeding intravenously through a small needle or tube inserted into an artery, or vein. There are three main types of intravenous lines: the umbilical artery catheter, the superficial IV and the central line. The umbilical artery catheter and superficial IV were both previously discussed.

A central line is a thick intravenous tube/long cannula that may be placed in one of the baby's larger veins, such as an arm, leg, scalp or neck. This type of IV is used when a baby needs IV fluids for an extended period of time. The central line can be placed in the vein through a small hollow needle. Once the tube is in place the needle is removed. The line may also be inserted by a minor surgical technique performed by a pediatric surgeon. Under a local anesthesia, a tiny incision is made over the baby's vein and the tube is threaded through the vein until it reaches a position as close to the baby's heart as possible. This procedure allows the IV line to be placed in a large central vein, which allows higher concentrations of nutrients and medications to be given. As your baby matures and grows stronger, this method of feeding will not be necessary. In the meantime, it allows your baby to receive the best nourishment possible.

Gavage (Tube) Feedings

Generally babies don't have the knowledge or even energy to suck for feeds till they reach 32 to 34 weeks and even if they do, they may not be sustained and coordinated, which leads to the risk of the baby getting food into the lungs called "aspiration pneumonia". Hence when extremely premature babies progress, they will be switched to gavage feedings, commonly referred to as tube feedings. Tube-fed babies have a small flexible tube inserted through their mouths or noses that passes down into the stomach or intestines. Since the transition from IV to tube feedings must be made gradually and carefully, there is usually an overlap period when the baby may receive both. Premature babies who have not yet developed a gag reflex do not seem to find the gavage tube uncomfortable. The tube may be left in place for continuous feedings or inserted and withdrawn for periodic feeds.

A gavage-fed baby is able to suck and has been doing so since the early months of gestation inside the mother's body. However, they can't learn to feed from a nipple until they learn to suck, swallow, and breathe in the right order. Because sucking is a very import activity for your baby, gavage-fed babies are sometimes given pacifiers to suck during their gavage-feedings, or they prefer to suck on their fingers on their own tongues. Sucking is an activity that babies enjoy and often find consoling. As gavage feeding is increased, IV feeding is decreased and stopped altogether once the baby is receiving enough calories by gavage.

Your baby's first gavage feed is usually breast milk for a day or two. Then, if all goes well, your baby may be given donor breast milk or formula if there is not enough breast milk. Many mothers may find it difficult to produce enough milk in the first few days to couple of weeks as their body may not be ready to produce enough milk due to premature birth. Your baby can receive breast milk that you have pumped (called Expressed Breast Milk – EBM) and taken to the NICU.

Breastfeeding

If you had planned during your pregnancy to breastfeed your baby, you don't have to give up the idea just because your baby is in the NICU. The milk that comes in the first few days after you give birth is especially good for your baby. It's called colostrum and it contains disease fighting substances called antibodies.

Breastfeeding a premature baby is usually divided into two stages. During the first stage, breast milk is pumped or expressed and fed to a baby by a gavage tube or by paladai or by a bottle. During the second stage, the baby is taught to suck from the breast. Since it may be a while before your baby can nurse from your breast, it's very important to pump your breasts to stimulate milk production. You can pump or express milk with a breast pump. There are several types of breast pumps on the market. The battery and electric types of pumps are the easiest for mothers to use. At Cloudnine we have breast pumps available for your use while you're in the hospital. You can discuss the same with the nurse-in-charge of the NICU or the lactation consultant when you visit the baby.

For a newborn baby you should pump at least six to eight times a day, with one of these pumping being at night. Any milk that you produce can be saved and given to your baby. Your NICU staff will discuss the guidelines for pumping, storing and transporting your breast milk with you. If you have any question about how to pump your breast milk,

discuss them with the NICU nurses. They can get you started
or refer you to an expert who can help you.

Sometimes a substance called a fortifier, such as Human
Milk Fortifier, is added to your breast milk to provide the
extra nutrients that your premature baby may need.
Remember, even if your breast milk is being given to your
baby by bottle or paladai or tube feeding, you can still
successfully breastfeed and in time your baby will be ready to
nurse from your breast.

Latching on

To feed from your breast, your baby will need to learn the
right way to latch on to your nipple. By latching on
correctly, it will be easier for them to get enough milk
and it will also be more comfortable for you.

To latch on properly, your baby should hold your nipple
firmly between its tongue and the roof of the mouth. To get
your baby to latch on, lightly touch the center of their lower
lip with your nipple. They will open their mouth as if they are
searching for it. This is called rooting reflex. Place your
nipple on the top of its tongue and guide it toward the back
of the roof of its mouth. Our NICU staff/Lactation
consultants will be there to teach you all these.

Many premature babies need to be wrapped snugly to feed
well. They should be held in a way so that the head, neck and
back are in alignment and have good support. The first
feedings may only involve licking and mouthing of the nipple
as the reflex to suck may be weak. Your baby's feeding skills
will improve as they get stronger and can stay awake longer.

Formula feeding

If you are unable to breastfeed, or decide not to do so or not to use donor breast milk, your baby will receive infant formula with your consent. Although breast milk is recommended, you can still feel confident that your baby is receiving excellent nutrition from infant formula. There is no need for you to be worried about bonding with your baby, as holding your baby, touching, talking to him/her, making eye contact, and feeding will allow the two of you to bond and become close.

Tips for Feeding - Waking to Feed

If your baby is asleep when it's time for a feeding, wake him/her by gently stroking arms and legs. Be patient. It may take five minutes or so to become alert enough to eat. If they are still sleepy, you might try changing his/her diaper to help them wake up.

When they start to look awake, begin talking to them. Tell them it's time to eat and say their name. Try saying You must be hungry by now, or You're a hungry little baby, aren't you? Tell him/her you love them and say whatever comes naturally. When they're awake, pick them up and cuddle them or you can do KMC/KFC. Hold them so that they can see your loving face.

Let your baby suck and eat at its own pace. Don't try to rush them by moving the nipple around in its mouth. They will determine their own natural rhythm of sucking and swallowing, breathing and resting. If they suck without stopping to take breaths, remove the nipple from their mouth every so often and set the baby up so they can catch their breath.

If the baby coughs or chokes while feeding, then the baby

needs to take a break. At first, the feeding process may be a little overwhelming for your baby and you. You can let the baby start sucking again when it has calmed down. Our NICU nurses are trained to help you with all these issues. They will be standing next to you till you get the confidence to do it all by yourself.

When to end the feeding

When your baby begins to lose interest in eating, its probably time to end the feeding. The baby will let the nipple fall out of his/her mouth, and the whole body may become relaxed. If this happens sooner than 15 or 20 minutes into the feeding, your baby may not be full and should be encouraged to finish the feeding. From start to finish, the feeding shouldn't take much longer than 30 minutes. If you try to feed much longer, your baby is likely to get tired and you both may feel frustrated.

How quickly your baby learns to suck properly and feed will vary. Just be patient. There is no standard guideline or timetable as each baby is different. When you first begin to feed, don't expect the baby to look at you, watch your face or pay much attention to you at all. The baby may be too busy learning how to feed. If you have any questions or concerns about feeding, don't hesitate to ask your NICU nurse. Remember: Persistence, Perseverance and Patience (3 Ps) are the three tools required to teach your puny infant to feed!

Learning to Feed

*   When I was_____days old, I had my first tube feeding.

*   It consisted of _____

*   I nursed (or took a bottle) for the first time when I was _____ days old.

Here I am on _____

```
┌─────────────────────────────────────────┐
│                                           │
│                                           │
│                                           │
│              BABY PHOTO                   │
│                                           │
│                                           │
│                                           │
└─────────────────────────────────────────┘
```

*   The first person to feed me was
    _____

*   When I graduated from tube feeding to nursing (or bottle feeding), my chart said I weighed _____ grams.

MILESTONES IN DEVELOPMENT

Development is a term that refers to the ways in which an infant matures and learns new skills, if your baby had stayed in the womb until your due date, the development would have continued there until the baby was ready to be born. But because it arrived early, he/she still has some developing to do. This is the reason the baby's age doesn't match the size, weight or the things the baby should be able to do. Because of these things, you can't compare your baby to a full-term baby who was born at about the same time. To adjust for this gap, we define a **corrected age** we calculate the age of any baby born prematurely in terms of weeks i.e. if a baby is born at 32 weeks and is 2 weeks old, we say the baby is of the corrected age of 34 weeks and so on. This we do till the age of 2 years and is more important for babies born at less than 32 weeks, especially when one is assessing developmental mile stones.

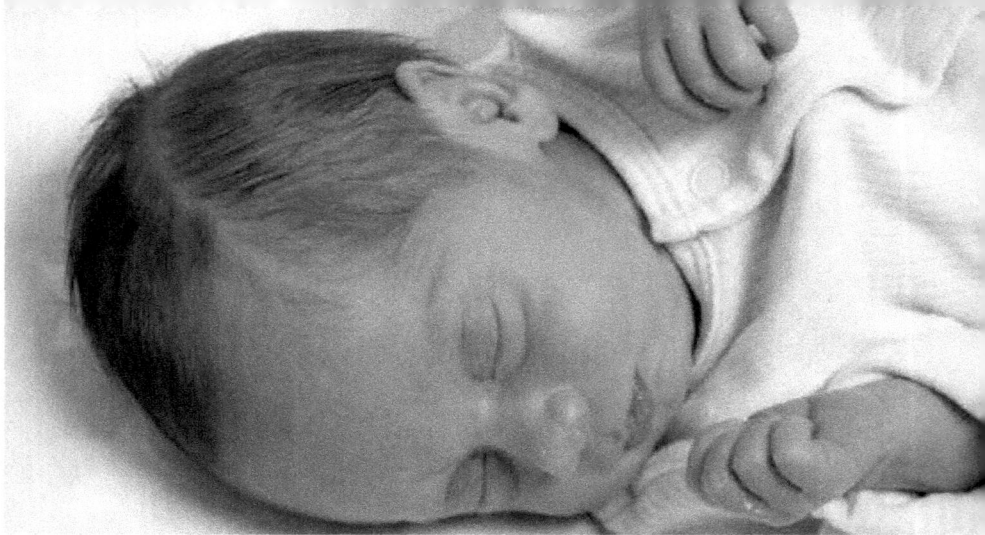

Don't worry, in time your baby's development will catch up. Recent studies have shown that most premature babies do as well as other children once they have had a few months to grow and mature. Remember, that no two babies are alike. One may progress faster in one area, but take longer in others; this is especially true if you are having twins!

Thus, your baby's development will progress in very small steps. Every day the baby is learning to gain control over his/her body in ways that full-term babies are born knowing and do automatically. Your baby's nervous system controls how well the vital organs function. Because the nervous system is still maturing and developing, the heart rate, breathing, nerves and muscles aren't working properly yet. The stronger the baby grows, the more signs you will see that their nervous system is gaining control. Below we have listed some milestones in development that you will notice in your baby as they develop. A developmental pediatrician is available in all Cloudnine Hospitals, who will follow your baby's development and assess the baby at fixed intervals.

- Heartbeat: Your baby's heartbeat will become regular and grow stronger as they grow. They will no longer need medicines to help in regulating their heartbeats. Till 34 weeks some babies may need a medicine called caffeine to regulate their breathing and heart rate.

- Breathing: Your baby's lungs will mature and develop, and will no longer need machines, such as a ventilator or CPAP to help him breathe.

- Digestive System: As your baby's digestive system matures, they will progress from IV feeding to tube feedings and eventually to breast or bottle-feeding.

- Muscle Control: As your baby's nervous system develops, they will gain better control of the muscles in their arms, legs, and the entire body. The movements will become smoother and they will be able to make the muscles do what they want them to.

- Regular Sleeping and Waking Patterns: Since premature babies require so much sleep, it may be hard for your baby to be wide awake and pay attention to what's going on around him/her. Soon though, waking and sleeping patterns will be more like those of a full-term baby. As your baby grows, you will be able to better predict their waking and sleeping patterns. They may sleep anywhere from 15-20 hours per day. Soon enough they will be alert, able to grab your finger or hair, and give you that unforgettable first smile.

IS THE BABY NORMAL?

One of the first questions that most parents ask after the birth of their baby especially when preterm is, "is the baby all right, other than being preterm?' Immediately after birth, even though the baby is preterm they are examined for any abnormalities such as anything that is underdeveloped (taking into consideration their prematurity) or something which shouldn't have developed, and for any evidence of problems / injuries caused by the actual process of being born (birth trauma). The baby is always given a score for his condition at one minute and five minutes respectively after birth. This is called 'APGAR' score – which is based on that Activity, Pulse (Heart rate), Grimace, Appearance (Colour) and Respirations (breathing). This is a score which lot of parents worry about. It is a score intended for the doctors to "attend to" if need be rather than anything else. If there is a concern, a further score is carried out at 10 minutes and that is worth noting, as it will give an indication of any ongoing problems with development.

Clinical examination

Soon after birth ALL babies @ Cloudnine will be examined from top to bottom for any abnormalities and also a tube is passed through the nose to ensure the passage is fully developed and open, and also from the bottom to ensure the anus is open.

On the morning after delivery the baby is given a thorough clinical examination again. She is checked again; the doctor listens to the heart, looks at the fontanelles (the two soft spots in a baby's skull), and the baby's hips are tested to see if they are loose or dislocated.

DDH

Developmental Dysplasia of Hips are one of the most important aspects in a new born baby – unfortunately many Indian parents are not even aware of this. All babies @ Cloudnine are checked for DDH. In the past it used to be called Congenital Dislocation of Hips (CDH) but now we know these hips are developing in the first 18 months hence it is nowadays called Developmental Dysplasia of Hips (DDH). Dislocated/Subluxated hips are probably the most important abnormalities to detect as early treatment is simple and generally effective. For every baby with a true dislocated hip that is detected and treated (with a splint) we find 20 with "clicky" hips (which are probably harmless) and have to ask the parents to bring the baby back for a repeat examination. This may seem very annoying for parents but hips are so important that it is better to be safe than sorry. If these hip problems are not detected at birth or within the first 18 months – then when they reach around 30 years of age, they could cause problems with hip pain or requiring hip replacement at an early age etc.,

All's well

If all is well the doctor may not discuss the routine screening examination with you and may not mention odd marks like bluish / greenish marks on the buttocks, or many things which are normal. Ex: There are normal birthmarks called Mongolian Spots that fade in time. Even so if you notice something that you are not happy about – don't forget to ask the doctor.

Counselling with Paediatrician

It is well recognised that prenatal and preconception counselling with a multi disciplinary team may be helpful in providing information to the family and to improve the standards of the care that can be provided to the couple during and after the pregnancy.

While there are no known guidelines that inform us about when the referral to the paediatrician is to be made, particularly preconception the following has been in practice. This therefore is not an exhaustive list.

Preconception counselling with paediatrician is advised for:

1. Previous child with developmental delay
2. Previous child with a known syndrome
3. Previous neonatal death
4. Previous child with known / suspected metabolic disease.

Involvement of a geneticist and a metabolic disease specialist may be needed in some instances.

Antenatal counselling with paediatrician

1. Babies with renal tract abnormalities, significant cardiac abnormalities, cranial abnormalities such as venticulomegaly, skeletal defects, congenital infection or any disorder noticed on Fetal Medicine Scan

2. Babies suspected of having haematological abnormalities (rising Rh titres, maternal thrombocytopenia, previous sibling with neonatal alloimmune thrombocytopenia).

3. Counselling with a pedaitric surgeon and pediatrician - may be desirable when surgical malformations like congenital diaphragmatic hernia, omphalocele, esophageal atresia, etc. are noted.

Pre-delivery counselling

1. Imminent preterm delivery
2. High risk consent for less than 28 weeks gestation delivery

TRANSFERS

Sometimes, depending on your hospital context, babies are transferred from Cloudnine to a step down nursery, where it is quieter and there are fewer machines. If you live far away from the NICU, your baby may be transferred to a hospital nursery near your home. The transfer will be discussed with you in advance and will occur only after the neonatologist, your local doctor and you agree that the transfer is appropriate. In most cases, the transfer will take place by ambulance.

If your baby is transferred, don't be surprised if you experience anxiety. Leaving a familiar place where you are comfortable and have adjusted is often hard. Just remember, even if they do things a little differently, your baby's new care providers are just as concerned about their well-being as the NICU staff. Give yourself time to get used to the new faces and surroundings.

72

GOING HOME

Each NICU will have its own guidelines regarding the discharge of your baby from the hospital. Listed below are some of the most common ones:

- Your baby will be able to control their own body temperature and keep warm without the help of an incubator.
- They will be able to breathe on their own, without the aid of a ventilator. (However, on rare occasions, some babies are allowed to go home on oxygen.)
- They can be breastfed or fed from a bottle.
- Their medical condition is stable. They weigh around 1500 grams or more, and are gaining weight at a steady rate.

Although we know you are very happy that your baby is going home, we understand that you may be a little nervous as well. This is completely normal. Don't worry, your NICU staff will not send you home unprepared. The NICU nurses are trained to help you get ready and guide you as you

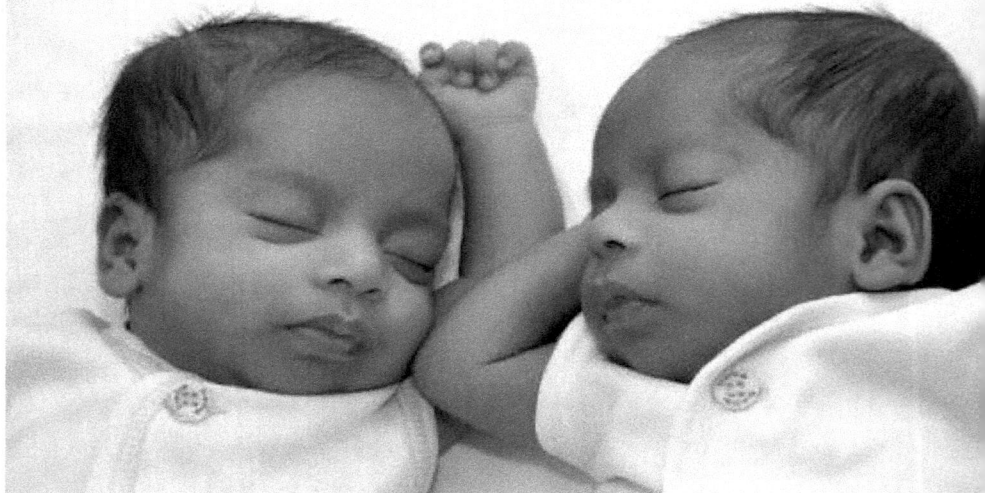

practice your baby's daily routine before taking him/her home. The nurses will help you bathe your baby and change diapers. They will coach you while you breastfeed and answer all your questions about feeding. The nurses generally know more about these things than the doctors, as they are the ones who do it every day!

They will also teach you how to take your baby's temperature and watch for signs of illness. If your baby is going home on oxygen or wearing some type of monitor, they will show you how to use it and monitor. They will instruct you about the use of any medications as well.

While your baby is still in the NICU, it is a good time to take a course in infant CPR (cardiopulmonary resuscitation). This life-saving course will teach you how to get your baby's heart and lungs working again if they should ever stop for any reason. Chances are you won't ever need to use CPR on your baby, but knowing it will increase your confidence and could save your baby's life. As a routine, we in Cloudnine teach CPR to all parents before their babies are discharged from the NICU.

Taking your baby home is a big step, but we know you can handle it! Spending as much time as possible with your baby in the NICU before going home will help you later. The staff will do everything they can to make the transfer to home the wonderful event that you have been waiting for! We generally recommend that you spend a night or two with the baby alone or with your partner in the room for mother/parent- crafting to see how you can cope and get a reality check and clarify any doubts.

On the following pages we have provided a pre-discharge checklist to help you remember everything you might need or want to know before going home, and a final list of discharge questions to help make sure you have covered everything you wanted to.

IMMUNISATION

Immunisations for your baby – PLEASE READ to understand your baby's vaccinations before discharge.

Vaccinations are important for babies to be protected against vaccine preventable diseases (VPD) which can kill them or cripple them. But babies generally who are born premature, especially less than 1000 gms, may get their vaccines delayed. Generally, any baby who is more than 1500 gms and 34 weeks, may be given vaccines similar to term babies. But premmie babies, the vaccines may be delayed a bit to help ensure they can tolerate them and also their immunity from the vaccinations is better. For example: at birth all babies are given BCG (for protection against TB), Oral Polio Vaccine (OPV) and Hepatitis B vaccine (HBV). In babies who are born premature, they are generally given when they are about to go home or discharged to improve their response to the vaccinations.

Tuberculosis is a serious disease. BCG is a vaccine that is given to protect children from severe forms of TB. This is the only vaccination given between the layers of skin – intra-dermally (that means between the layers of the skin – this is the ONLY routine vaccine that is given intradermally) - so **healing takes 3 to 4 months** and during this time – the place where BCG is given – looks like a mosquito bite initially after a week or so, then like a small red swelling appears by the end of week 2 or 3 and then it occasionally looks like a pustule – filled with pus – but it is not painful and over the next few days/weeks, it will rupture – later leading to healing by a scar. It is not painful and does not cause any discomfort to the baby during all this time and nothing should be applied to the place either. Any such things or applications, may delay healing and also may reduce the immunity. In some countries like USA or Canada or Australia, where Tuberculosis is uncommon, BCG may not be given @ birth, but if you are living in India for few months or visit India frequently, then your baby should be given BCG.

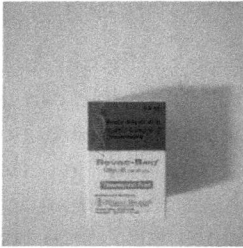

Hepatitis B attacks the liver. The virus is spread through blood to blood contact, sexual contact and sharing needles or sometimes through saliva through kissing. Prevention is with hepatitis B injections. This is one of the vaccines – the first dose is given soon after birth – hence it has to be mercury free. At Cloudnine we always use ONLY mercury free hepatitis B vaccine – if need more information please discuss with your Paediatrician.

Pertussis (Whooping Cough) causes a severe lasting cough, difficulty breathing and sometimes death. Most mothers should have received dTap during their pregnancy, which should protect the babies in the first 6 weeks. Pertussis vaccination starts at 6 weeks of age. Prevention is with DTwP (whole cell) of DTaP (acellular) injections. Most parents think of DTaP as "painless" injections in India & DTwP as "painful" vaccine. They are not painless – there are less chances of side effects with DTaP than compared to DTwP, hence it is erroneously called as painless injections. If your baby is premature or has had severe reactions previously, we always recommend DTaP injections. Discuss about your choice of DTPw or DTPa for your Baby with the paediatrician, when you visit for the vaccinations.

Diphtheria is a painful infection that blocks the throat. It can cause death due to heart or nerve damage. Diphtheria has been virtually eliminated in most countries, but it is still very much prevalent in India. Prevent with DPT or dTap injections.

Tetanus is a deadly disease that causes muscle spasm and sometimes death. It occurs after cuts, breaks in the skin or burns. Prevention is with DPT injection, dTap and booster injections every 5 to 10 years throughout life.

Poliomyelitis is a serious diasease and can paralyse parts of the body including the throat. Fortunately, India has been free of Polio for the last few years. Prevention is with Sabin Oral (OPV) or injectable polio vaccine(IPV). The common question asked is – should we be giving Pulse Polio when the government does it. Pulse Polio vaccine is totally different from routine polio vaccination. "Pulse Polio" as the name indicates is a PULSE of Polio vaccine given to all the babies and children under 5 years of age to raise the immunity all at once, that is how the wild Polio disease is eliminated. Whenever there is a threat of polio the government gives a "booster" immunity protection to all children under 5 years of age and this should be given to all children irrespective of their immunizations before or their regular vaccines they have received from their Paediatrician. India is at cross roads now, we have been FREE of polio infection for the last few years and if we are free of polio for few more years, then we will probably stop polio drops (required for gut immunity, as polio spreads by faeco-oral route) and give all babies Polio injections. The current recommendation is to give your baby

BOTH polio drops and polio injections for better protection as per the schedule printed in your book.

Haemophilus influenza type B causes meningitis and other childhood infections. Prevent with Hib injections. Hib meningitis is known to cause deafness, blindness or mental retardation in affected children. It is mandatory even by the government now.

Measles causes a red blotchy, flat rash. It can damage ears, lungs and brain. In the olden days, they used to have proverbs like "Count your children after measles" – that is how deadly the disease was supposed to be. Prevent it with Measles vaccine or MMR injection. Measles is re-emerging as a major problem in many countries. Please ensure your baby is well covered with measles vaccine.

Mumps causes swelling of glands, testicles and other important organs. Many affected boys can become infertile if they get mumps. Prevent with MMR injections.

Rubella (German measles) causes rash and fever. Women who have rubella early in their pregnancy are at risk of having a disabled or deaf baby. Babies may also be born with Congenital Rubella Syndrome (CRS). Women thinking about pregnancy should have a rubella test or prevent with MMR Injections.

Chicken Pox causes serious skin, eye and lung infections occasionally brain infection causing intellectual disability. Prevention is with Chicken pox vaccine. The first dose of Chicken pox vaccine is recommended after the antibodies from the mother disappears in the baby's body – which is generally around 1 year. Hence in Cloudnine we recommend the first dose of Chicken pox vaccine at 1 year – similar to USA – and a second does at around 4 years of age for lifelong protection.

Influenza causes fever, headache, sore throat, cough aches and pains. It can be life threatening for some people. Prevent with Influenza each year to at risk groups – generally children less than 5 years and grandparents or even parents with underlying medical conditions. Protection from FLU vaccine is for that year only and it needs to be given every year based on the WHO antigen recommendation. It is highly recommended for young babies and people older than 60 years of age.

Hepatitis A can cause serious jaundice + liver disease and in some children (and older adults) it can be fatal. 2 doses of the vaccine will protect your children from this deadly disease. Hepatitis A vaccine is recommended routinely even in countries like USA. The second dose of the vaccine should be given AFTER 6 months of the first dose but before 18 months (preferably around 12 months after) the first dose for life long protection.

Typhoid Disease Typhoid is a serious disease that causes lot of morbidity and mortality in India. It is still an endemic disease in India and one dose can prevent Typhoid in your child with vaccinations. Previously it was given every 3 years after which they need a booster does to protect them again, as they were polysaccharide vaccine. Currently (at the time of printing this book Nov 2020) the recommendation was to give the first dose anytime after 6 months and probably a booster dose after a year or two for protection over 15 years - but this is early and things can change in the future as lot of research is happening in this area.

Pneumococcal Infections are a serious threat to children under 5 years of age or for people above 50 years of age. It causes pneumonia, meningitis ("brain fever") and a lot of other serious infections in children, which can kill them or cripple them. Protect your child from this serious disease by vaccination with Pneumococcal Conjugate Vaccine (PCV) –

there are currently 2 vaccines available in the world and is mandatory in most developed countries because of its benefit. The first one is called Prevenar13 (Wyeth) containing 13 serotypes and the second one is called Synflorix (GSK) containing 10 serotypes – they cost Rs. 3,805 or Rs. 1,499 per dose respectively at the time of printing of this book and you will have to chose one of them for your baby and your Paediatrician can advise more details if required.

Rotavirus affects rich and poor equally by causing vomiting and diarrhea – hence it is called a **Democratic virus**! In serious cases it can cause death due to severe dehydration. Thanks to the vaccines we can protect our children from this deadly virus. At the time of printing this book there are 4 brands of this vaccine – Rotarix (GSK, UK) – 2 doses required; Rotateq (MSD, USA); Rotasure or Rotavac (Bharat Biotech, India) & Rotasiil (Serum Institute of India) – 3 doses for complete immunization. The choice of the vaccine is entirely left to the parents – but the brands should not be generally interchanged for better protection. WHO has pre-qualified all these vaccines for routine use.

Other optional vaccines are: Meningococcal vaccine, Japanese B encephalitis vaccine, Rabies vaccine, Yellow fever vaccine, and cervical cancer vaccine. If you need more information on these, please discuss with your Paediatrician.

At Cloudnine we keep a record of all the vaccines given to your baby including the batch numbers, which may be required at times. Also we use vaccines without mercury as per international norm, if you have any further questions, don't forget to ask your paediatrician.

Also it is important to note that the vaccines need to be stored in a particular temperature ALL the times. India being a developing country, there are power failures and also power fluctuations – please ensure that wherever you get the vaccines, they have enough power back up to protect the vaccines, otherwise the vaccines may be useless!

Premature babies' response to vaccinations are similar to term babies when administered as per your Paediatrician recommendations who will obviously follow the international consensus.

BEFORE GOING HOME

Before the exciting journey home, take a few minutes to review the checklist below. Its best to use this section several days before your baby's discharge date, so that if there are things you still need to ask about or do, such as take a CPR class, there will still be time before going home. We also suggest that all parents attend the Cloudnine MBA (Management of Baby Affairs) course at least 1 week prior to discharge, which would help you become confident parents.

I AM:

- Comfortable giving my baby a bath.
- Comfortable taking care of my baby's umbilical cord.
- Comfortable feeding my baby.
- Comfortable giving him/her medicines.

I:

- Know how long to breastfeed or how much to feed.
- Know how to mix the infant formula, if required.
- Know how to take an axillary (underarm) temperature and how to read the thermometer
- Know how to perform a CPR on my baby if necessary.
- Have clothes for my baby to wear at home.

● Things I would like/need to do prior to discharge:

_____

_____

_____

_____

● Final instructions from the NICU:

_____

_____

_____

_____

● NICU Phone Number: _____

● Notes:

_____

_____

- Graduation Day

- I graduated from the NICU on _____ (date) I was _____ weeks old

- I weighed _____ grams.

- I went home wearing _____

- My mom and dad were so proud!

Here's how I looked

BABY PHOTO

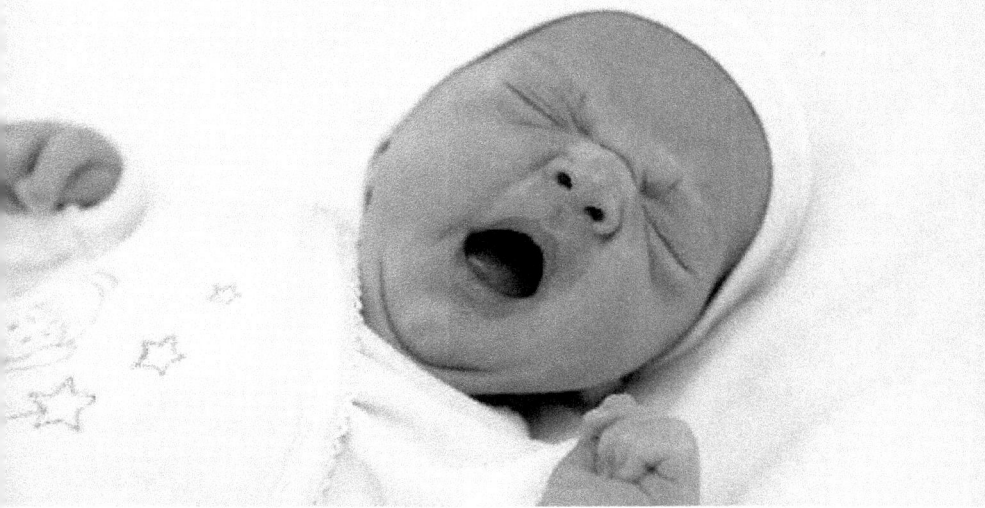

Hospital Visiting Guideline

Here is a handy place for you to jot down your hospital's visiting guidelines, as well as your baby's first visitors.

Visiting Hours: _____

Special Guidelines for Parents: _____

Grandparents: _____

Brothers & Sisters: _____

Others: _____

Other guidelines or Notes: _____

Baby's first visitors

Name

Date

FOLLOW UP FOR NICU BABIES

Baby's name: _____

Hospital No: _____

Mother's name: _____ Age: _____

Education: Professional / Matriculate / <10th.

Occupation: _____

Father's name: _____ Age: _____

Education: Professional / Matriculate / <10th.

Occupation: _____

Address:

_____

_____

_____

Gestational age: _____ EDD: _____

Birth weight: _____

Neonatal diagnosis and major interventions:

1. _____

2. _____

3. _____

4. _____

5. _____

PROCEDURE / INVESTIGATION	REPORT				ACTION REQUIRED
Neurosonogram					
ROP					
Hearing	AABR	R		L	
	BERA	R		L	

MRI		
Echocardiogram		
Other		

VLBW GROWTH CHART

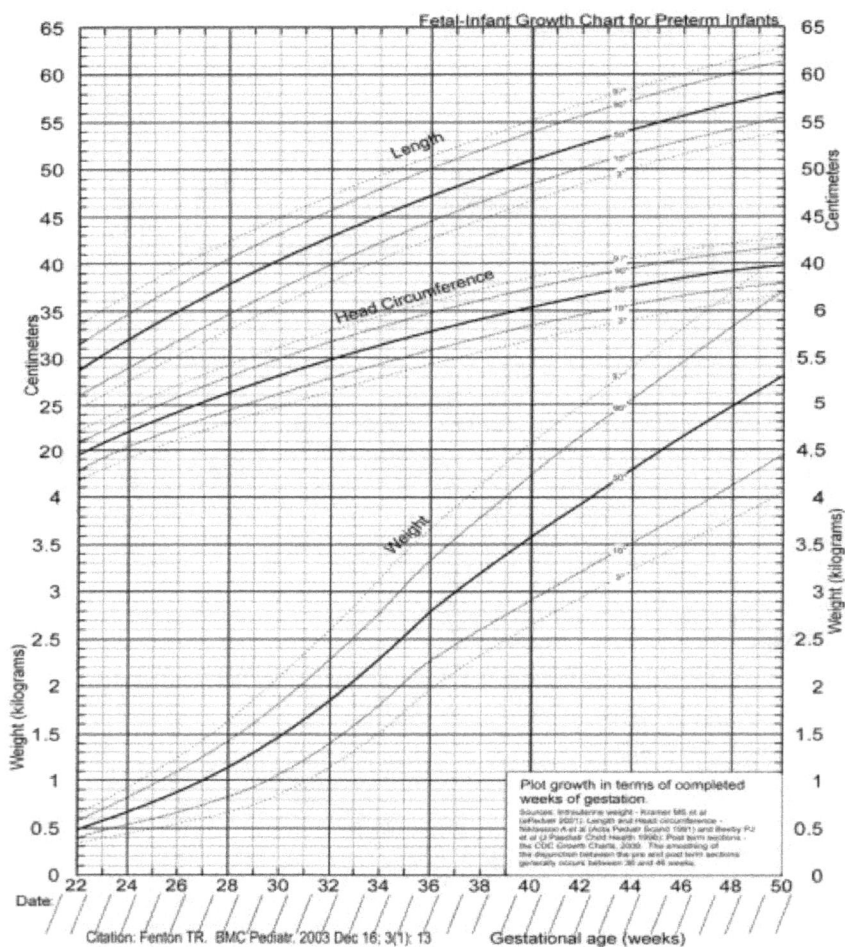

Fetal-Infant Growth Chart for Preterm Infants

Citation: Fenton TR. BMC Pediatr. 2003 Dec 16; 3(1): 13

Gestational age (weeks)

Plot growth in terms of completed weeks of gestation.

NEURO-DEVELOPMENTAL FOLLOW UP

What is neurodevelopmental follow up?

Neurodevelopmental follow up is a systematic way of tracking your baby's development at regular intervals. Ideally, all babies should be followed up. This is more important in the case of babies born prematurely, with low birth weight, with birth defects, with Downs Syndrome and in those who suffered fits, or required intensive care for any reason at or soon after birth.

What happens at these follow up visits?

At follow up visits, your baby's growth parameters are monitored, developmental history is taken, and developmental screening and examination are performed. Parental guidance is given to facilitate normal development in your baby.

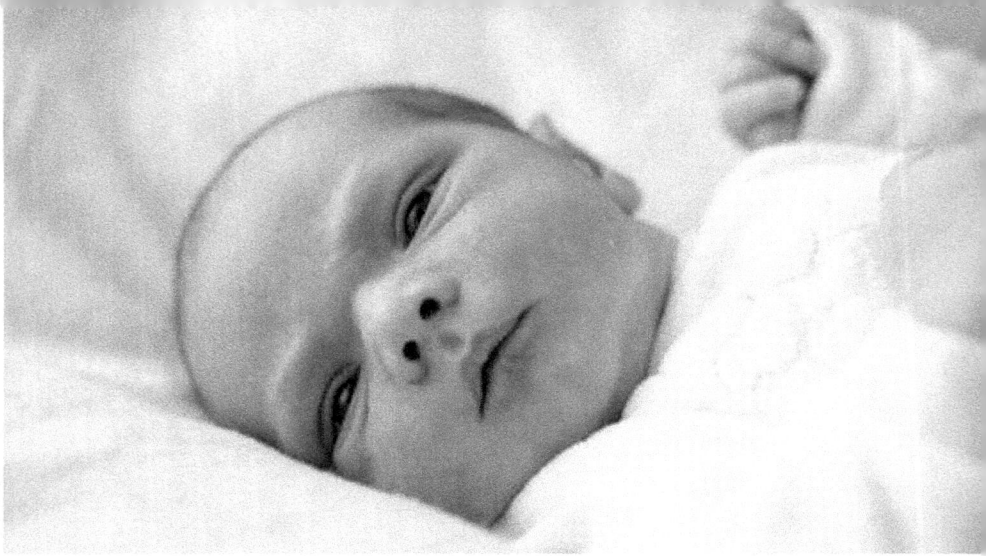

How frequent are these visits?

Premature babies are examined once at their expected date of delivery, and then at 2 months, 4 months, 8 months and 12 months in the first year. Thereafter, they are screened at 6 month intervals until they start formal schooling.

Why is this necessary?

It is necessary because prematurity, low birth weight and certain illnesses are considered high risk factors, which means these factors may delay the baby's development in one or more areas. In order to detect these delays early and to start corrective steps, regular monitoring is essential. Delays may manifest or become detectable only as the child grows and may not be identifiable in the early stages.

Do all high-risk babies have developmental delays?

No, majority of the babies do not have developmental delays, but some may have mild developmental delays. A small percentage of babies will have more significant delays.

What is developmental assessment?

Developmental assessment is a way of formally assessing your baby's development in all domains namely gross motor, fine motor, speech and language, socio-emotional and general understanding. The assessment helps us understand your child's development and areas of strength and weakness. This will enable us to chart out a program of activities to catch up in those areas of weaknesses. Assessment is important in high risk babies. Usually it is done at the first year mark of corrected age.

If the baby is found to have a developmental delay, then what will be the next step?

The next step is to start the baby on an 'Infant stimulation program' with the objective of minimizing delays and facilitate catching up. This may involve physiotherapy or other activities which have to be carried out regularly at home. This will be based on the developmental assessment.

DEVELOPMENTAL CHECKLIST

0 - 4 MONTHS	4 - 7 MONTHS
MOVEMENT Raises head and cheek when lying on stomach (3 mos.) Supports upper body with arms when lying on stomach (3 mos.) Stretches legs out when lying on stomach or back (2-3 mos.) Opens and shuts hands (2-3 mos.) Pushes down on his legs when his feet are placed on firm surface (3 mos.)	**MOVEMENT** Pushes up on extended arms (5 mos.) Pulls to sitting with no head lag (5 mos.) Sits with support of his hands (5-6 mos.) Sits unsupported for short periods (6-8 mos.) Supports whole weight on legs (6-7 mos.) Transfers objects from hand to hand (6-7 mos.) Uses raking grasp (not pincer) (6 mos.)
VISUAL Watches face intently (2-3 mos.) Follows moving objects (2 mos.) Recognizes familiar objects and people at a distance (3 mos.) Starts using hands and eyes in coordination (3 mos.)	**VISUAL** Looks for toy beyond tracking range (5-6 mos.) Tracks moving objects with ease (4-7 mos.) Grasps objects dangling in front of him (5-6 mos.) Looks for fallen toys (5-7 mos.)
HEARING AND SPEECH Smiles at the sound of voice (2-3 mos.) Cooing noises; vocal play (begins at 3 mos.) Attends to sound (1-3 mos.) Startles to loud noise (1-3 mos.)	**LANGUAGE** Distinguishes emotions by tone of voice (4-7 mos.) Responds to sound by making sounds (4-6 mos.) Uses voice to express joy and displeasure (4-6 mos.) Syllable repetition begins (5-7 mos.)

0 4 MONTHS	4 7 MONTHS
SOCIAL/EMOTIONAL Begins to develop a social smile (1-3 mos.) Enjoys playing with other people and may cry when playing stops (2-3 mos.) Becomes more communicative and expressive with face and body (2-3 mos.) Imitates some movements and facial expressions	**COGNITIVE** Finds partially hidden objects (6-7 mos.) Explores with hands and mouth (4-7 mos.) Struggles to get objects that are out of reach (5-7 mos.)
VISUAL Watches face intently (2-3 mos.) Follows moving objects (2 mos.) Recognizes familiar objects and people at a distance (3 mos.) Starts using hands and eyes in coordination (3 mos.)	**SOCIAL EMOTIONAL** Enjoys social play (4-7 mos.) Interested in mirror images (5-7 mos.) Responds to other people's expression of emotions (4-7 mos.)

Corrected age	4 Months				8 Months			
Date								
Popliteal								
Adductor								
Heel to Ear								
Ankle dorsiflexion								
Scarf sign								
Muscle tone:	UL	LL	Neck	Trunk	UL	LL	Neck	Trunk
DTR	UL		LL		UL		LL	
CDC grading head control								
CDC grading sitting								
Vision: strabismus/ nystagmus / other								
Response to hearing:								

Developmental screening

Domain	4 Months	8 Months
Gross motor		
Language		
Fine motor adaptive		
Personal social		

Next follow up on:

1. _____

2. _____

3. _____

8 - 12 MONTHS	12 - 24 MONTHS
MOVEMENT Gets to sitting position without assistance (8-10 mos.) Crawls forward on belly Assumes hand and knee position Creeps on hands and knees Pulls self up to standing position Walks holding on to furniture Stands momentarily without support May walk two or three steps without support	**MOVEMENT** Walks alone (12-16 mos.) Pulls toys behind him while walking (13-16 mos.) Begins to run stiffly (16-18 mos.) Walks into ball (18-24 mos.) Climbs onto and down from furniture unsupported (16-24 mos.) Walks up and down stairs holding on to support (18-24 mos.)
HAND AND FINGER SKILLS Uses pincer grasp (grasp using thumb and index finger) (7-10 mos.) Bangs two one-inch cubes together Puts objects into container (10-12 mos.) Takes objects out of container (10-12 mos.) Pokes with index finger	**HAND AND FINGER SKILLS** Scribbles spontaneously (14-16 mos.) Turns over container to pour out contents (12-18 mos.) Builds tower of four blocks or more (20-24 mos.)
COGNITIVE Explores objects in many different ways (shaking, banging, throwing, dropping) (8-10 mos.) Finds hidden objects easily (10-12 mos.) Imitates gestures (9-12 mos.)	**COGNITIVE** Finds objects even when hidden under covers (2 -3 nos.) Begins to sort shapes and colors (20-24 mos.) Begins make-believe play (20-24 mos.)

LANGUAGE MILESTONES Responds to simple verbal requests Responds to no Makes simple gestures such as shaking head for no Babbles with inflection (8-10 mos.) Babbles dada and mama (8-10 mos.) Says dada and mama for specific person (11-12 mos.)	**LANGUAGE** Points to object or picture when it's named for them (18-24 mos.) Recognizes names of familiar people, objects, and body parts (18-24 mos.) Says several single words (15-18 mos.) Uses two-word sentences (18-24 mos.) Follows simple, one-step instructions (14-18 mos.) Repeats words overheard in conversations (16-18 mos.)
SOCIAL/EMOTIONAL Shy or anxious with strangers (8-12 mos.) Cries when mother or father leaves (8-12 mos.) Enjoys imitating people in his play (10-12 mos.) Shows specific preferences for certain people and toys (8-12 mos.) Prefers mother and/or regular care provider over all others (8-12 mos.) Repeats sounds or gestures for attention (10-12 mos.) Finger-feeds himself (8-12 mos.) Extends arm or leg to help when being dressed.	**SOCIAL / EMOTIONAL** Imitates behavior of others, especially adults and older children (18-24 mos.) Increasingly enthusiastic about company or other children (20-24 mos.) Demonstrates increasing independence (18-24 mos.) Begins to show defiant behavior (18-24 mos.) Episodes of separation anxiety increase toward mid-year, then fade.

NEONATAL COMPLICATIONS

This book will be incomplete without writing a bit about complications of prematurity and death. I am sure no one would like to talk about the adversities, but the reality is that these things do happen.

As a general rule,

Late preterm   34+0 to 36+6 weeks do very well. They have higher chance of having jaundice, feeding issues and some may need to stay in the hospital for few days more or may need to be readmitted for treatment of jaundice or feeding issues. Most babies will do well, without major problems.

Preterm   32+1 to 33+6 weeks – generally most survive to the extent of 90 to 100%. Most babies will need to stay in the NICU for 2 to 4 weeks depending upon each baby.

Moderate Preterm babies born between 28+1 to 32 weeks. The average survival for this gestation is anywhere up to 80% and above in most centres with good NICU. Majority of the babies in this group do well, with a minority having developmental problems. Most babies will need spend anywhere between 4 to 6 weeks in the NICU before discharge.

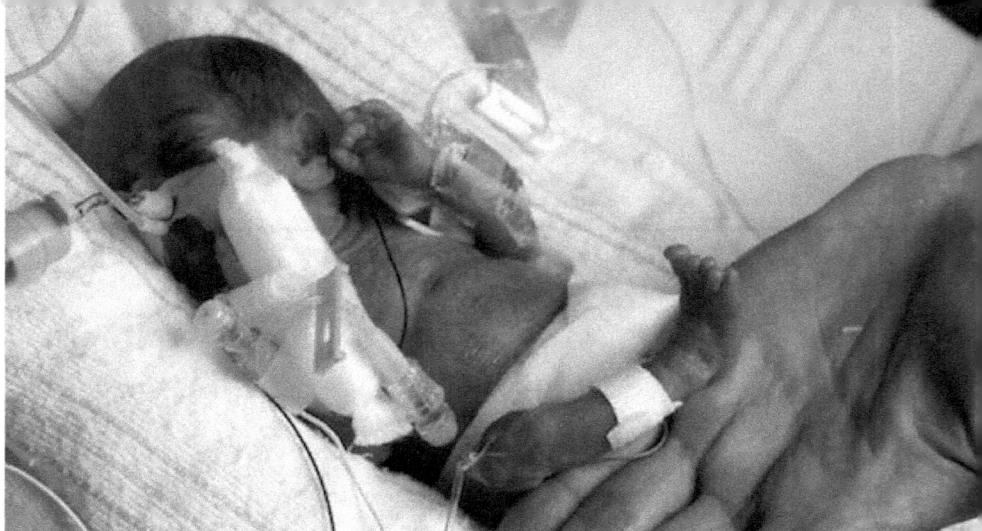

Extreme Preterm babies born between 24 weeks to 28 weeks. Survival for this group of babies could vary from 50 to 75% depending upon various factors. 10 to 20% of babies could have developmental problems depending upon what complications they develop during their first few weeks of life. *Each day in the womb is equal to 1 week outside, is what we generally say.* Most babies in this group land up needing to spend 10 to 12 weeks in the NICU before getting discharged.

This is NOT a comprehensive list or a text book to discuss about all complications or adverse effects. In the chronological order the problems that could happen are as follows:

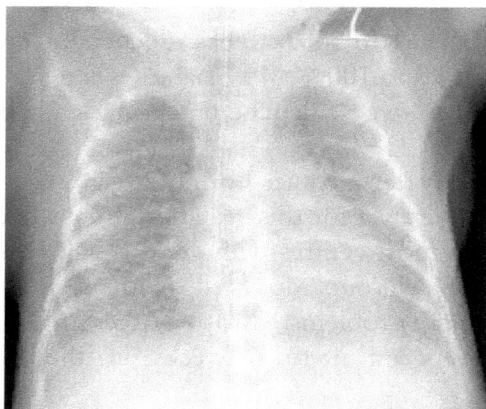

Respiratory Distress Syndrome (RDS) – Premature babies lungs are very stiff due to lack of a substance called surfactant which makes the lungs spongy. If the babies lungs are stiff, we need to give surfactant medicine into the lungs and also put the baby on ventilator or CPAP till the lungs soften and oxygenation happens easily. Generally babies need 2 doses of surfactant, if they are having RDS. Surfactant is a medicine that became available in early 1990s and the cost has been coming down steadily. Still it costs around Rs.6,000 per dose or could be lower if a synthetic surfactant, instead of a natural surfactant (which is better).

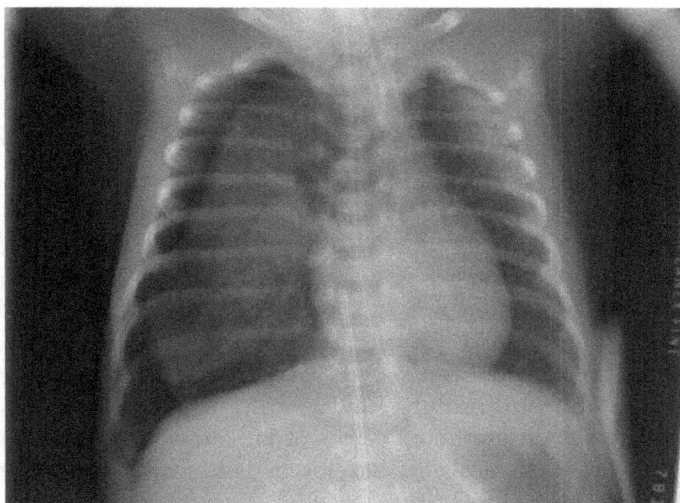

Pneumothorax – this is generally due to "mild tear" in the lungs causing air to accumulate in between the lungs and the chest wall. This has become rarer since surfactant treatment these days. But it is related to how stiff the lungs are. If this were to happen, your neonatologist will explain to you and baby will need a chest drain for few days to help the lungs expand.

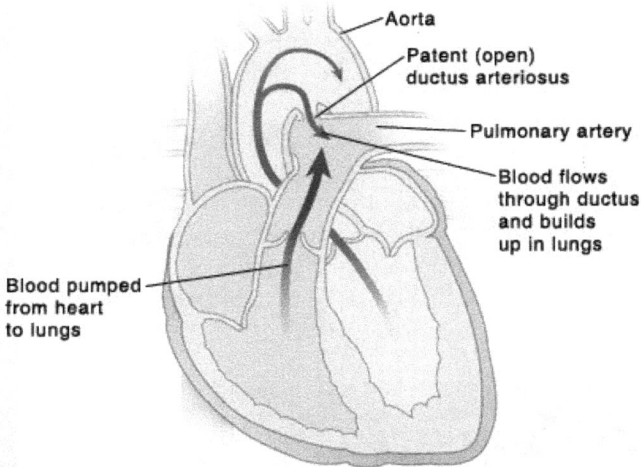

Patent Ductus Arteriosus (PDA) – Commonly called "duct" – this is basically a normal blood vessel called ductus arteriosus present in all babies and is expected to close soon after birth when the lungs get filled with air after the "fluid" is expelled and lung expands – but in some babies with RDS, this duct is kept open for various reasons or sometimes it opens up too causing congestion of lungs with "blood flowing" towards the lungs. This can sometimes cause trouble in some small babies with breathing as they feel "almost breathing under water". Generally this can happen anytime in the first 2 weeks of life and your neonatologist will tell you, if it needs to be closed with medications. Rarely surgery may be required, if it stays open and causes problems for long.

Sepsis – this is a word you will hear very frequently while your baby is in the nursery/NICU. Infection of the babies born premature is very common because the more premature the baby is much higher the risk of infection. Infection can happen commonly in babies because they don't have antibodies from their mothers because they are born premature and also they are susceptible for bacteria which commonly colonise adult bodies/hands – hence strict precautions are taken to avoid infection in babies. Sometimes babies can get infection from the germs in their intestines too. Infection is one of the common causes of babies get sicker and "going back" few days in their progress and sometimes it is one of the causes of death too in very sick very premature babies.

Anaemia – You will hear this word very often in preterm babies. The more premature the babies are the more likely they will develop anaemia – because of multiple reasons – the repeat blood tests will reduce blood in their body, their bones/body would not have started manufacturing new blood yet, they are deficient in iron stores (raw material required for red blood cells being manufactured) and so on. Extreme preterm babies generally need two or three blood transfusions before they go home. Every precaution is taken if your baby needs blood transfusion/s and your staff in NICU will explain well in advance the process that is followed, except in case of emergencies.

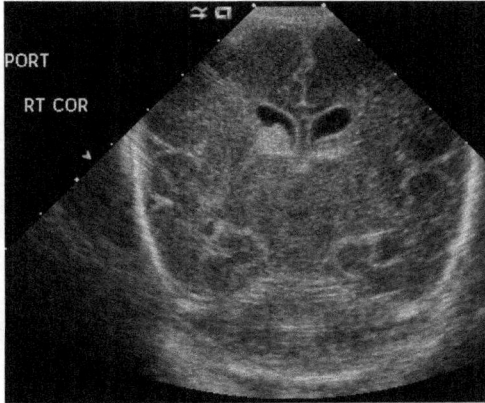

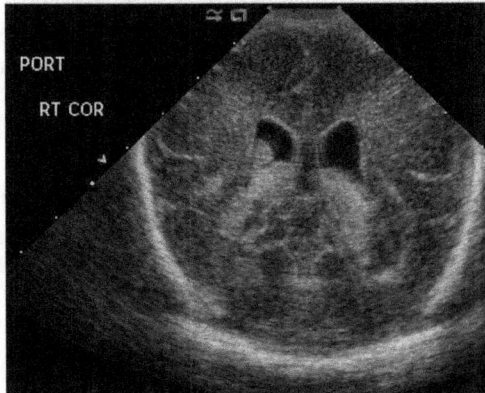

Intra-Ventricular Haemorrhage (IVH) – commonly known as IVH is brain haemorrhage in extreme preterm babies – can happen anytime but more commonly in the first week of life. The brain of preterm babies is very fragile – fluctuations of oxygen levels, or blood pressure or sometimes with just prematurity they can bleed inside. This can happen in the first week of life commonly. Most mothers who go into premature labour are treated with steroid injections, to reduce the chances of this happening. There are different grades of this described based on the extent of the haemorrhage, but generally grade 1 is not a major concern, though ideally no haemorrhage should be there. All preterm babies will have ultrasound scan of their heads to monitor for this in the first week and then after a month to ensure the brain is good. Rarely this can be so gross that it can be fatal in some extreme preterm babies.

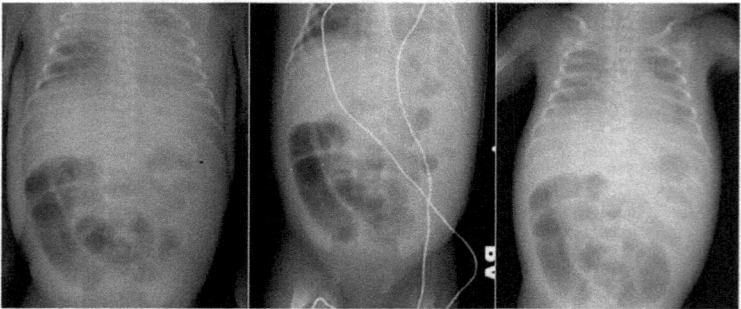

Necrotising Entero-Colitis (NEC) – is known commonly as NEC, is an uncommon but a dreaded complication of preterm especially of extremely preterm babies in the second to 4th week of life. The exact reasons why it happens in some babies and doesn't happen in others is not known. Suffice to say that it is an infection of the "gut" that leads to the gut rotting on itself and also causing gut perforations, leading to babies needing to "rest their guts" for 2 weeks and be treated with antibiotics for them to recover. Sometimes these babies require emergency surgery for the rotten gut to be removed or perforations to be closed to help them recover. Very rarely some babies die due to this complication, when everything seems to be going well, especially in extreme preterm babies. Every precaution is taken to reduce the chances of your baby developing this.

DEATH – this is a word no one likes to hear or talk about. But the reality is, NOT all preterm babies especially extreme preterm babies survive. Some babies could develop some complications which are beyond human endeavour to save them. In such unfortunate situations, your NICU team will talk to you of the steps involved and how to avoid such things for future.

DR. KISHORE KUMAR

IMPORTANT INFORMATION FOR MOTHERS

Breast Feeding best for the baby

Breast milk is a complete and balanced food and provides all the nutrients required by the baby for the first six months of life; thus minimizing the likelihood of excesses and deficiencies. Breast milk has anti-infective properties that protect the baby from the infections in the early months. Breast milk is always available.

Breastfeeding- best for the mother

Breast feeding is convenient. Breast milk needs no utensils or water (that might carry germs) or fuel for its preparation. When you are away from home, you wont need to carry formula, bottles and nipples. Breastfeeding immediately after delivery enables contraction of the womb and helps the mother regain her figure quickly. Mothers who breastfeed usually have longer periods of infertility after childbirth than non- lactators. Breast feeding gives you a special sense of closeness to your baby and can provide you with much emotional satisfaction.

Don't be afraid to ask for help

Breast feeding is not something you should know how to do just because youve had a baby. Nursing is a skill that takes some practise. Take help of a lactation consultation or hospital staff. Make sure that the hospital staff knows you want to nurse the baby as soon as possible after delivery.

The first food- Colostrum

Immediately after delivery, breast milk is yellowish and sticky. The milk is called Colostrum, which is secreted during the first week of delivery. Colostrum is more nutritious than mature milk because it contains more proteins and more anti-infective properties which are of great importance for the mothers defence against dangerous neonatal infections. It also contains higher levels of Vitamin A. Colostrum also helps the baby have her first bowel movements.

Formula feeding:

If you have any questions about your baby's diet, ask your baby's doctor .He or she is the best source of information regarding your baby's nutrition. If your doctor or any other healthcare professional recommends an infant formula in addition to breast feeding or its replacement during the first 4-6 months, keep the cost in mind before deciding whether to use infant formula. You will need more than one can (400gm) per week if your baby is only bottle-fed. Breastfeeding is much cheaper than feeding infant milk substitute as the cost of the extra food needed by the mother is negligible compared to the cost of feeding infant milk substitute.

Difficulties in reverting to breastfeeding

Infants fed on formula get accustomed to its taste. As a result, mothers may find it difficult to reverse their decision to feed infant formula. Partial formula feeding may hinder the restart of breastfeeding.

Management of breastfeeding

- Breastfeeding is successful when baby suckles frequently and the mother wanting to breastfeed is confident in her ability to do so.

- In order to promote and support breastfeeding, the mother's natural desire to breastfeed should always be encouraged by giving, where needed, practical advice and making sure that she has the support of all her relatives.

- Adequate care for the breast and nipples should be taken during pregnancy.

- It is necessary to put baby to the breast as soon as possible after the delivery.

- Let the mother and her baby stay together after the delivery. The mother and the baby should be allowed to stay together (in hospitals, this is called rooming-in).

- Give the baby colostrum as it is rich in many nutrients and anti-infective factors protecting the baby from infections during the first few days of its birth.

- The practice of discarding colostrum and giving sugar water, honey water, butter or other concoctions insteadof colostrum should be very strongly discouraged.

- Let the infant suckle on demand.

- Every effort should be made to breastfeed the baby whenever he/she cries.

- Mothers should keep her body and clothes and that of her baby always neat and clean.

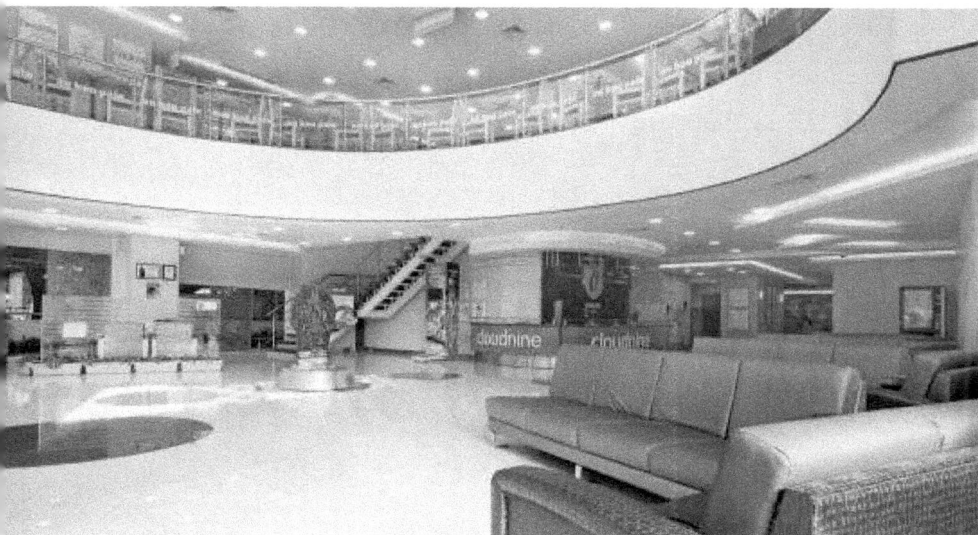

ABOUT CLOUDNINE

Driven by the core objective of delivering world-class healthcare services in India, Cloudnine healthcare facilities heralded the beginning of a new era for all woman and child care needs, especially for preterm babies. Cloudnine is the result of the founder, Chairman and senior neonatologist Dr. R. Kishore Kumar's vision of bridging the ever- widening gap between Indian and international standards of healthcare.

Since inception in 2007, innovation, integrity and quality have spanned our comprehensive portfolio of services offering Pregnancy, High Risk Pregnancy, Neonatal, Paediatric, Gynaecological, Infertility and Newborn Intensive Care.

With a diversified, well trained and motivated workforce, Cloudnine has achieved and sustained nearly zero percent maternal mortality rate and 99.2% survival rates for babies, despite the high risk cases we undertake. We are immensely passionate about what we do, and this has led to our success

115

as the leading provider of quality woman and child care in India.

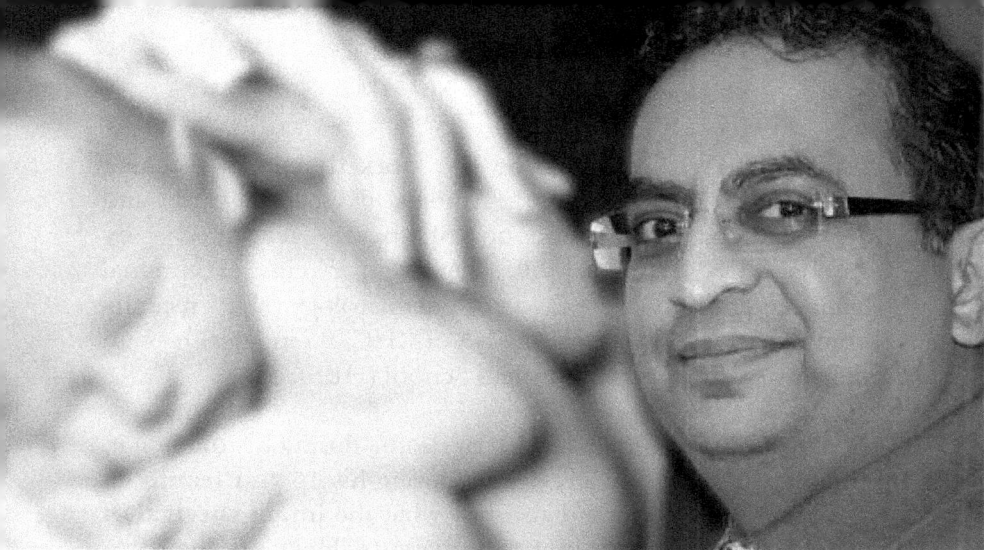

ABOUT THE AUTHOR

Dr. R. Kishore Kumar founded Cloudnine in 2007 to further his vision for bringing high quality maternal & neonatal healthcare to India, on par with international standards. He conceived the idea of a facility dedicated to providing exclusive and comprehensive services in maternal and child care. As the Founding Chairman, and senior neonatologist, he has been instrumental in securing the pinnacle of success achieved by Cloudnine today.

Dr. Kishore is an internationally acclaimed neonatologist who has worked in four continents over the course of his career including North America, UK, Asia and spent 12 years in Australia. He completed his MBBS from Gulbarga University and his DCH from Mysore University and London. Amongst his many qualifications, he also has an MD with a gold medal from Mysore University, MRCP (Paed) & FRCPCH from UK as well as MRCPI (Paed) and FRCPI from Ireland. He has also completed his Fellowship in the Advanced Neonatal ICU with an FRACP from Melbourne, Australia. At the time of his qualification, he was one of the youngest and highest qualified neonatologists in the world. To his credit, he has worked only in teaching hospitals around the world. Among his many awards and accreditations is the honour of being felicitated by former US President Bill Clinton for his exceptional achievements in the field of neonatology. He recently completed his executive MBA (MHCD) in health care delivery from Harvard Business School (HBS).

Dr. Kishore Kumar saw lot of deaths during his training in India, but hardly saw any deaths during his 16 year tenure in the developed world and also saw what the **intact survival** of a premature baby means to the parents. Hence he had this dream of providing similar care in India and is committed to his passion for scaling new heights in neonatology as he pioneers this modern concept of maternal healthcare in India with Cloudnine. To this effect, he has achieved more than what he dreamt for the Cloudnine group can boast of over 1000 deliveries a month, having nearly ZERO percent maternal mortality and 99.2% survival for babies including premature babies as premature as 24 weeks. These achievements led to several awards such as the Economic Times, Leaders of Tomorrow Award received in Dec 2012 from Mr. Anand Sharma, Commerce minister of India. Cloudnine also received the BEST Maternal and Neonatal Hospital Award for three consecutive years 2011, 2012 and 2013. He received Australian Service Excellence Award – the ONLY health care facility in India to have received this award. He was also bestowed with Pride of Karnataka award recently. He has also established teaching and research programmes of international repute and has published over 80 papers in national and international conferences in the last few years. These academic contributions led to Indian Academy of Pediatrics gold medal in 2012, FNNF by National Neonatology Forum of India and Fellow of Indian Academy of Pediatrics (FIAP) in 2018.